Textbook of

INDUSTRIAL PHARMACOGNOSY

Textbook of

INDUSTRIAL PHARMACOGNOSY

Anusuya R Kashi
Assistant Professor
Department of Pharmacognosy
Vivekananda College of Pharmacy, Bengaluru

S Ramachandran
Assistant Professor
Department of Pharmaceutical Chemistry
Mohamed Sathak AJ College of Pharmacy, Chennai

Bindu Sukumaran
Assistant Professor and Head
Department of Pharmacognosy
Vivekananda College of Pharmacy, Bengaluru

Universities Press

UNIVERSITIES PRESS (INDIA) PRIVATE LIMITED

Registered Office
3-6-747/1/A & 3-6-754/1, Himayatnagar, Hyderabad 500 029 (A.P.), India
info@universitiespress.com; www.universitiespress.com

Distributed by
Orient Blackswan Private Limited

Registered Office
3-6-752 Himayatnagar, Hyderabad 500 029 (A.P.), India

Other Offices
Bangalore / Bhopal / Bhubaneshwar / Chandigrah / Chennai / Ernakulam / Guwahati / Hyderabad / Jaipur / Kolkata / Lucknow / Mumbai / New Delhi / Noida / Patna

First published in India by
Universities Press (India) Private Limited 2012

ISBN 978 81 7371 754 3

Typeset in Life BT 11/13.6 *by*
OSDATA, Hyderabad 500 029

Printed in India by
Multifold, Chennai 600 085

Published by
Universities Press (India) Private Limited
3-6-747/1/A & 3-6-754/1, Himayatnagar, Hyderabad 500 029 (A.P.) India

Foreword

Today the world is moving from spiritual to digital. The digitization of herbal medicines, once considered spiritual, is progressing at a rapid pace. There is global resurgence in the use of traditional systems of medicine which are based on drugs of natural origin.

Knowledge of *Industrial Pharmacognosy* is essential for the effective use of medicines exclusively derived from natural sources. Industrial pharmacognosy deals with a process of social and economic change, which is in turn a part of a wider modernization process, closely related to technological innovation, particularly with the development of large-scale production of drugs of natural origin.

As a practicing pharmacognosist, an educationist and member of the Board of Studies for undergraduate and postgraduate studies in pharmacy, I have felt the need for a standard textbook in the field of industrial pharmacognosy, suitable for the Indian educational system.

I am happy that three young pharmacognosy teachers have come out with a very useful book on industrial pharmacognosy. I am sure this book will be an invaluable guide to the budding pharmacognosist and congratulate the authors and the publisher for the student-friendly, attractive and easy-to-refer layout of this book. I recommend that the authors bring out regular editions of this book, updating the latest developments in the field. I also hope the book will motivate readers to admire and appreciate Nature and highlight natural remedies.

Prof. V Gopal
Academic Registrar,
Mother Theresa Post Graduate and Research Institute of Health Sciences,
A Govt. of Puducherry Institution,
Puducherry

Preface

Scientific research on herbs used in traditional medicine has gathered momentum, promising results in the treatment of a wide range of diseases and disorders. At the same time the herbal drug industry is faced with the challenge of designing safe and effective formulations.

The current scenario of the herbal drug industry is significantly different from what it used to be as recently as a decade ago. Herbal medicines are not new to India; the increasing demand for quality herbal products—both within the country as well as abroad—is however recent. Just as it is important to verify the therapeutic efficacy of drugs used in traditional medicine, it is also necessary to use modern manufacturing and analytical techniques to ensure the preparation of herbal products of standard quality. This, along with the applications of plant biotechnology, forms the bulk of the subject matter of *Industrial Pharmacognosy*.

As teachers with more than a decade's experience in teaching this subject, we realized that there is no single book that provides both contemporary *and* comprehensive information on herbal drugs. Therefore, we began with the premise that this book has to be different from others in two aspects: it should provide the latest information, and be organized in a format that enables students to focus on the important aspects.

While the book represents a refined version of lecture notes prepared from well-known texts in the field of pharmacognosy, a substantial portion of the information is new and has been culled from diverse sources, including reliable websites, the details of which are provided in the bibliography at the end of the book.

This book is designed for undergraduate pharmacy students and covers the syllabus prescribed by Rajiv Gandhi University of Health Sciences, Karnataka, and MGR Medical University, Tamil Nadu, for the third and final year BPharm course.

The chapters have been grouped as follows:

- Herbal drug industry, intellectual property rights, patents and WHO guidelines for standardization
- Alternative systems of medicine, methods of preparation of herbal formulations, quality parameters and drugs used in traditional medicine
- Isolation, identification and estimation of certain secondary metabolites
- Role of herbs in cosmetics
- Nutraceuticals
- Plant biotechnology dealing with enzyme biotechnology, polyploidy, protoplast technology and genetic transformation.

Throughout the book, it has been our endeavour to use a student-friendly approach. The learning objectives at the beginning of the chapter and the summary at the end help reinforce the concepts covered in the chapter. We understand that students look for not merely knowledge of a subject, but also an orientation towards what is important from the examination point of view. This led us to provide a list of questions for each topic that have appeared in university examination papers till date.

We have sought to check and verify every detail provided in this book. Yet, it is possible that some errors may have found their way in. We will be greatly obliged if readers bring these to our notice.

We trust that students will find this a useful book that helps them grasp the relevance of industrial pharmacognosy. In addition and perhaps, more importantly, we hope that reading this book instils a sense of pride in students for belonging to a land that has such a rich heritage and knowledge of traditional medicine. We also hope that the book will motivate readers to support and protect this knowledge from loss and misappropriation by those who seek to patent that which should be freely available for use by all.

To express in written form that which you effortlessly teach in a classroom is challenging, to say the least. Writing this book has been a demanding, yet immensely fulfilling, experience. We thank our families and friends for their support and encouragement, which made it possible for us to take up and complete this project. We are grateful to our college authorities for providing access to the library facilities during the course of our research for the book.

We sincerely thank Prof. Gopal for agreeing to provide the Foreword. We would also like to place on record our gratitude to Ms Javanthi Singaram of Universities Press for her patience and guidance at every stage of the process. We are also grateful to Dr KK Balasubramaniam, Retd Professor, Department of Chemistry, IIT Madras, Chennai, for his encouragement to write this book, and all the help and support he has rendered.

We would like to thank Dr PK Warrier, Arya Vaidya Sala, Kottakal, for granting us permission to use the botanical sketches from Warrier PK, Nambiar VPK and Ramankutty C, *Indian Medicinal Plants: A Compendium of 500 Species*,Vols 1–5, Universities Press, Hyderabad, India, 1996. All the images in the colour plates have been sourced and reproduced from *Wikipedia Commons* (http://commons.wikimedia.org) under the terms of the GNU free documentation license. We acknowledge our gratitude to this website, which has remained an ever-bountiful source of a vast collection of images under every category.

Anusuya R Kashi, Ramachandran S, Bindu Sukumaran

Contents

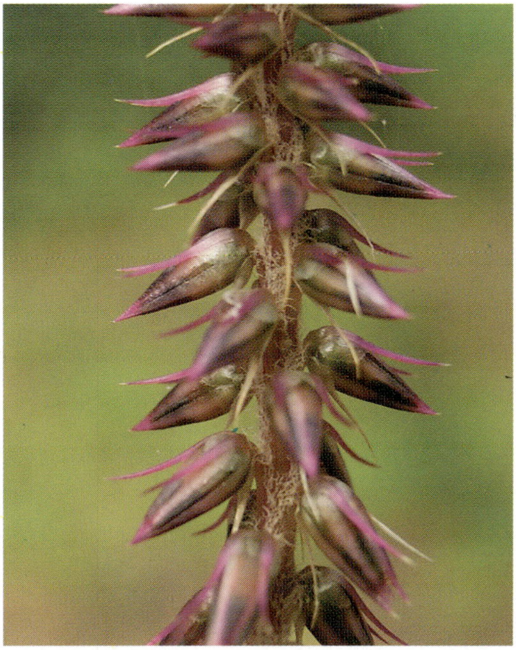

Apamarga
Achyranthes aspera

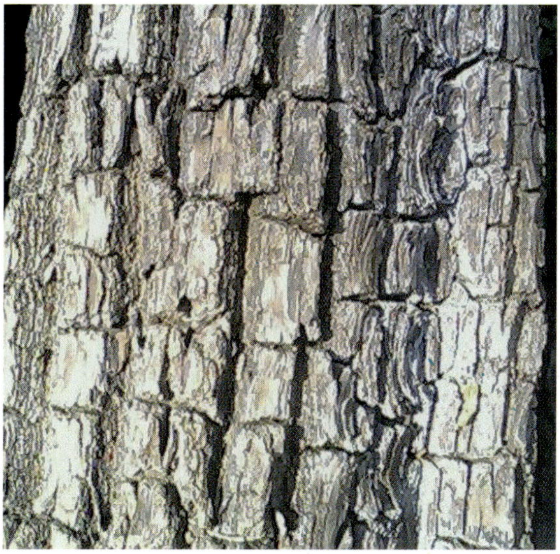

Arjuna (bark)
Terminalia arjuna

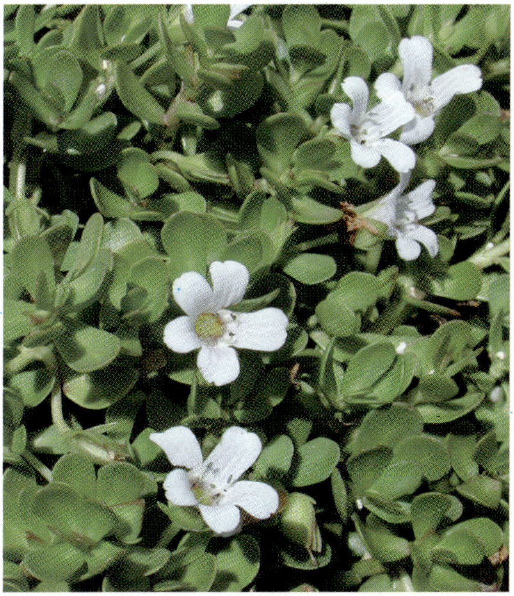

Brahmi
Bacopa monieri

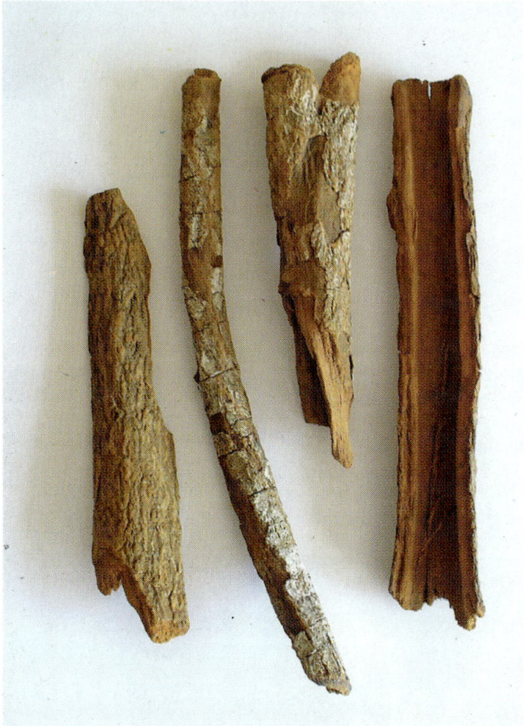

Cinchona (bark)
Cinchona officinalis

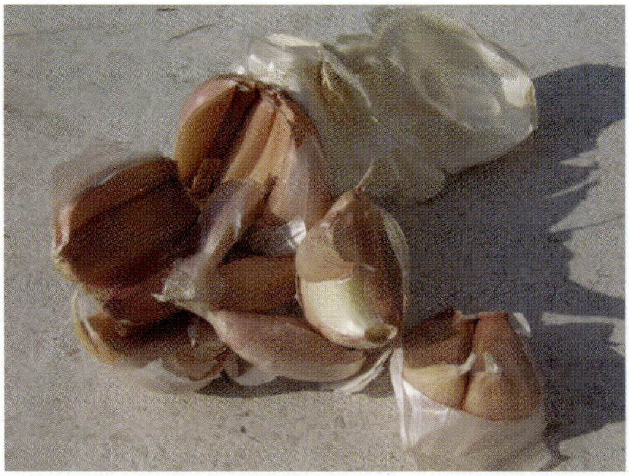

Garlic
Allium sativum

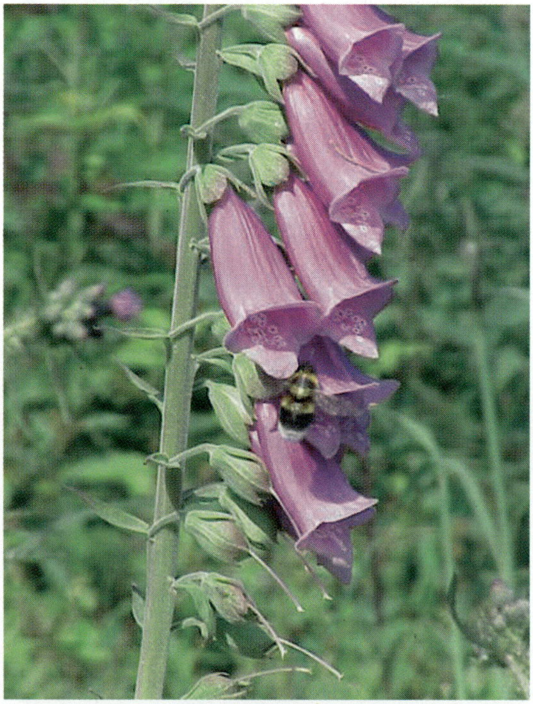

Foxglove
Digitalis purpurea

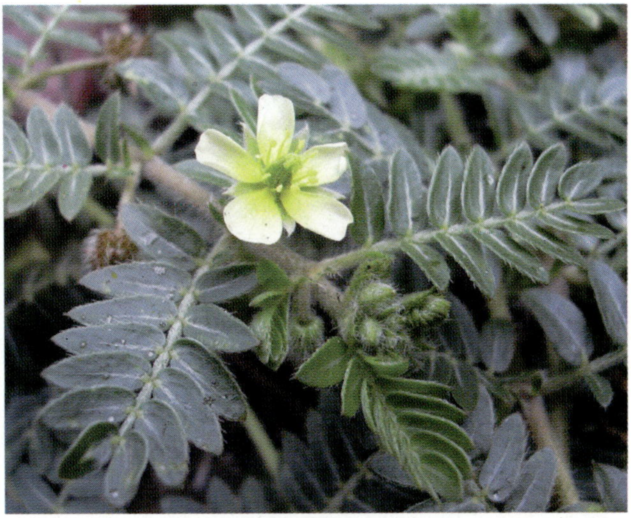

Gokhru
Tribulus terrestris

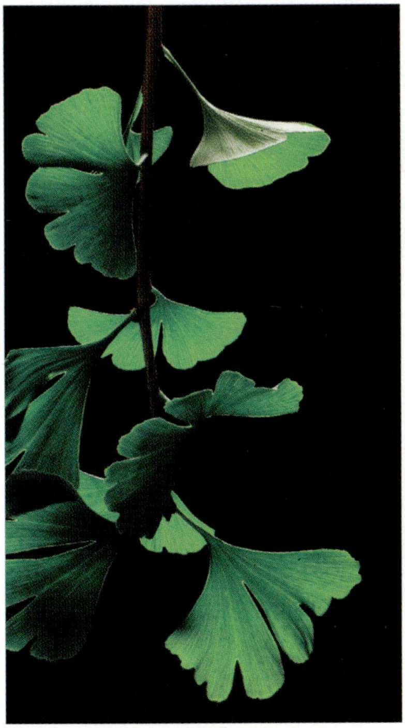

Ginkgo
Ginkgo biloba

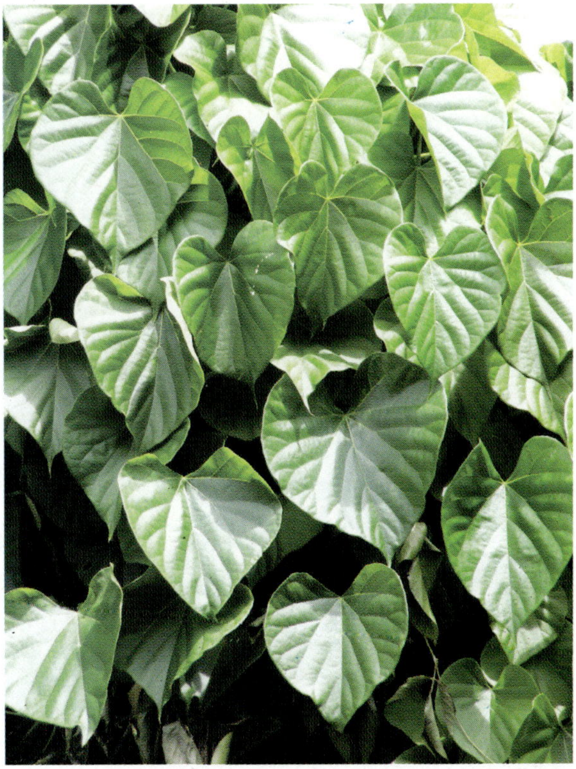

Guduchi
Tinospora cordifolia

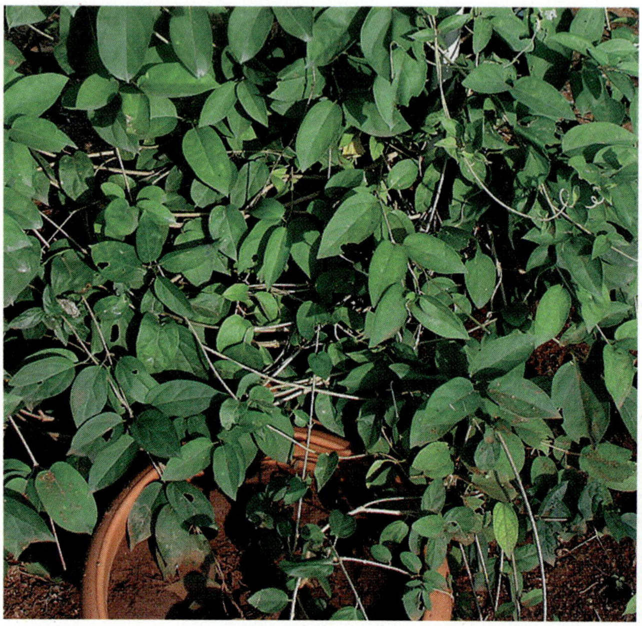

Gurmar
Gymnema sylvestre

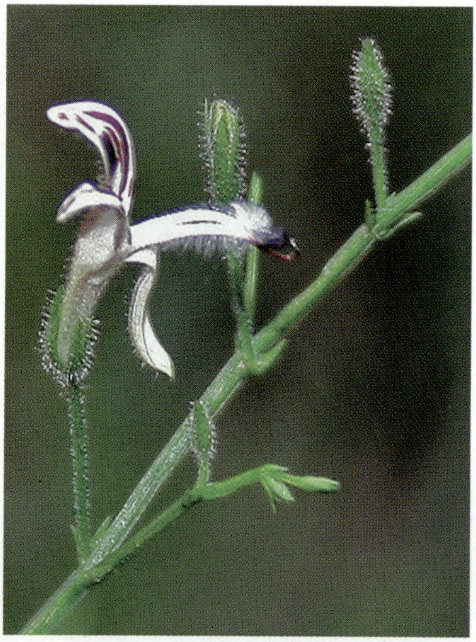

Kalmegh
Andrographis paniculata

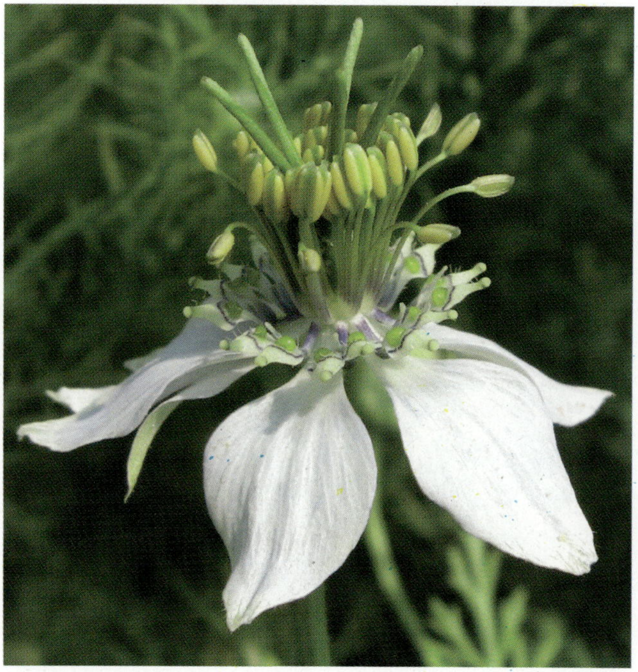

Kalijeera
Nigella sativa

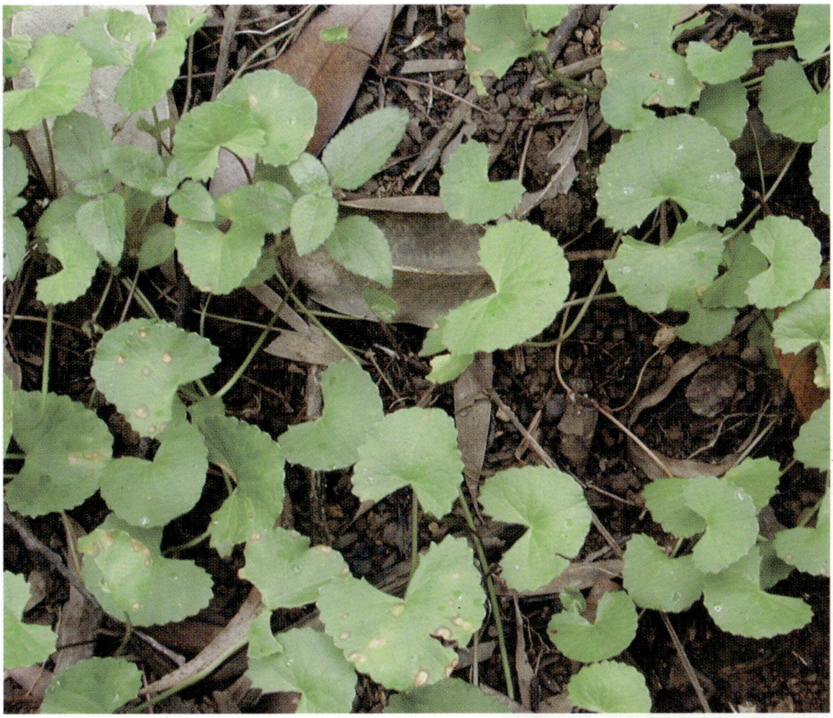

Mandukaparni
Centella asiatica

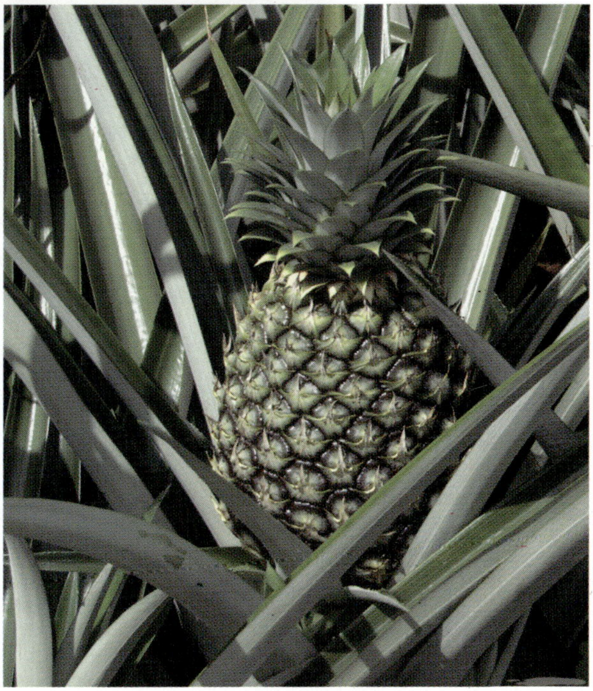

Pineapple
Anana comosus

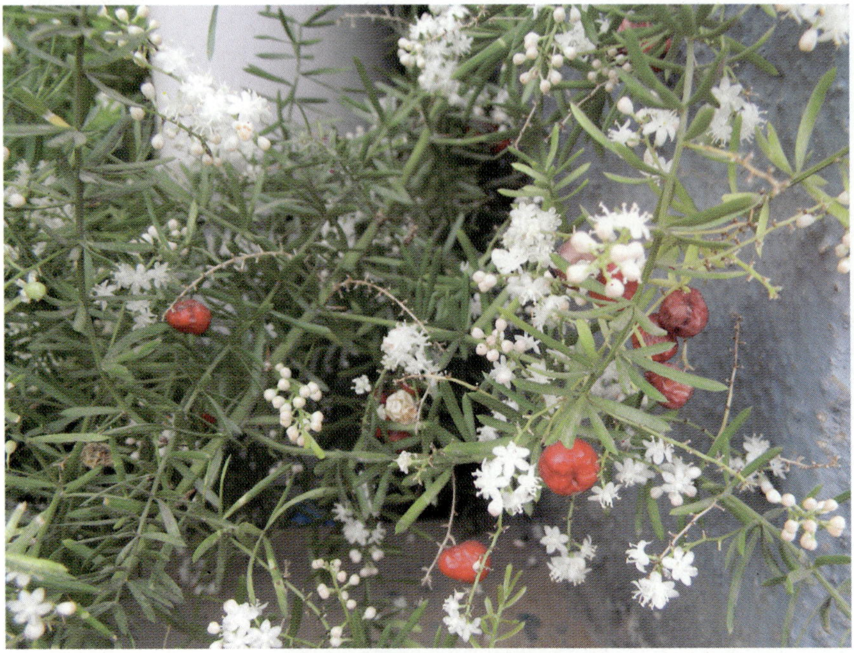

Satavari
Asparagus racemosus

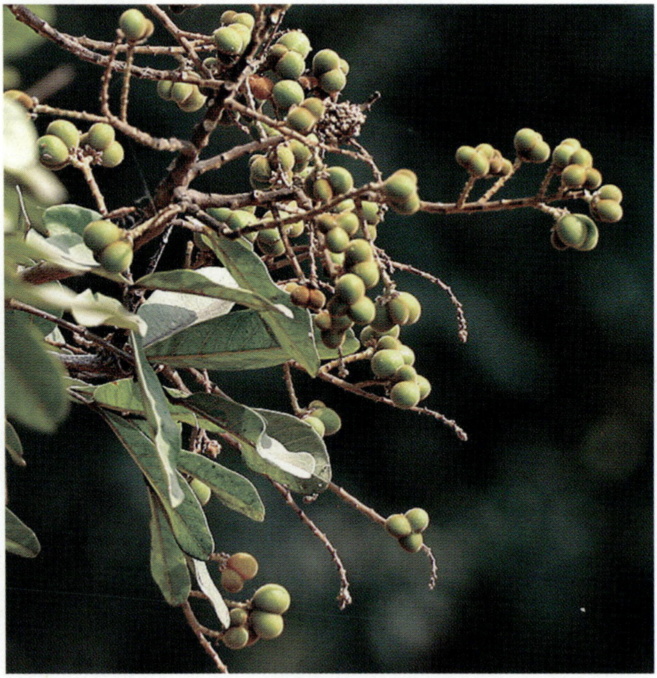

Soap nut
Sapindus marginatus

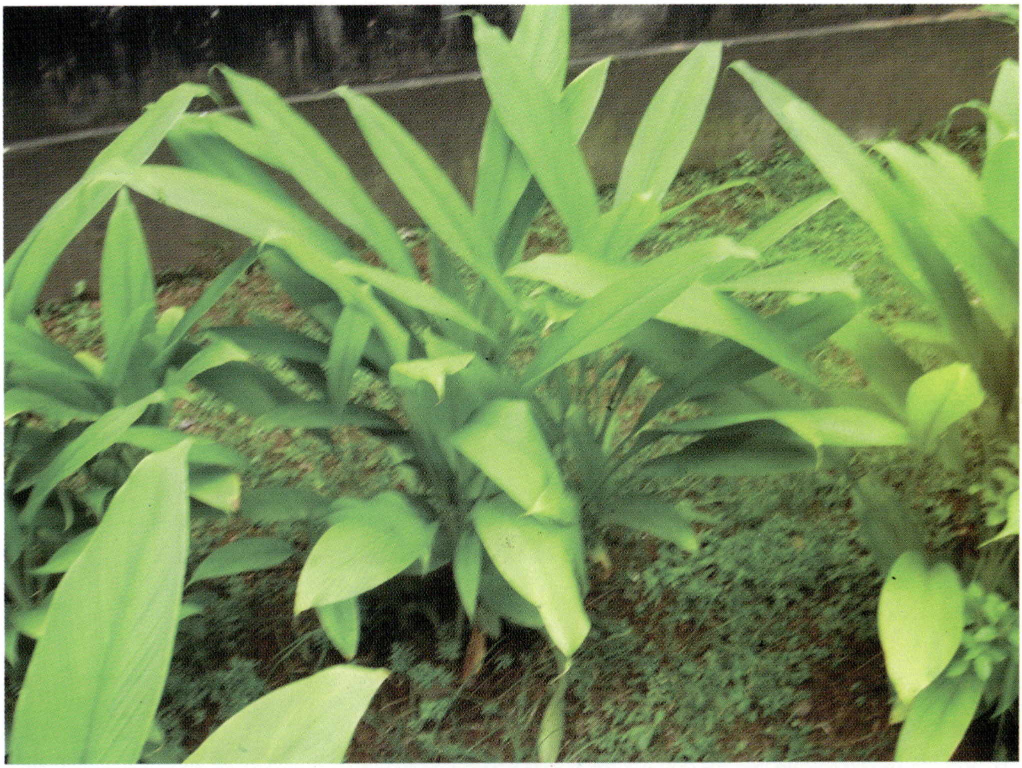

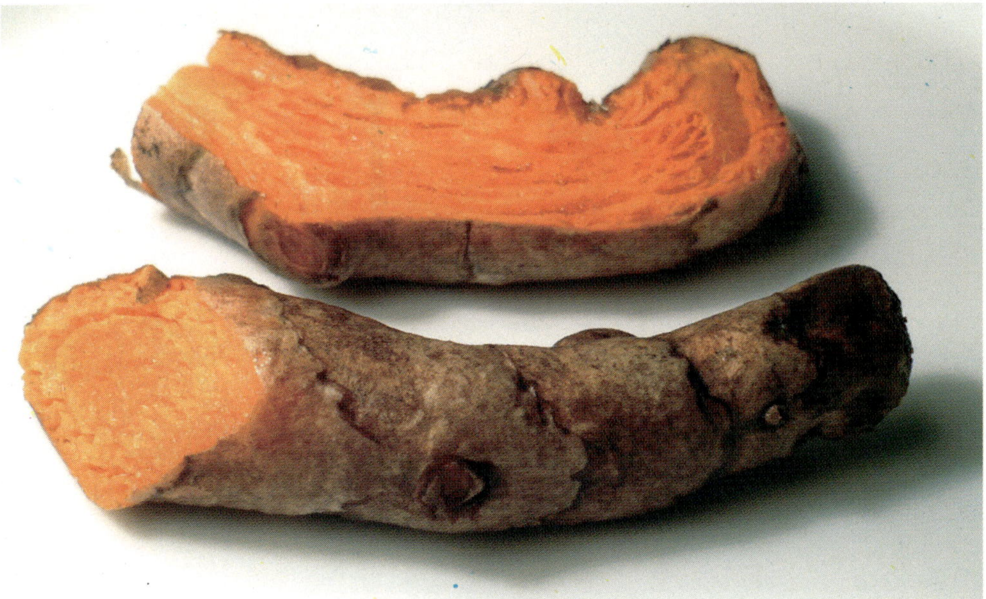

Turmeric (plant and rhizome)
Curcuma longa

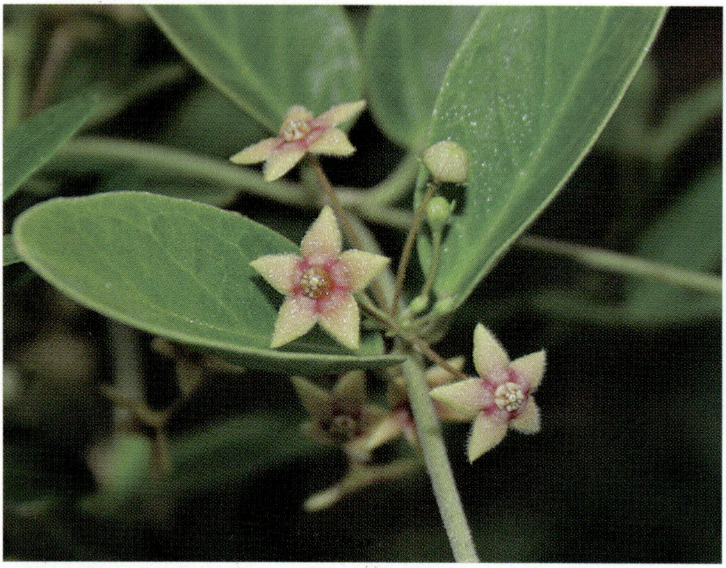

Tylophora
Tylophora indica

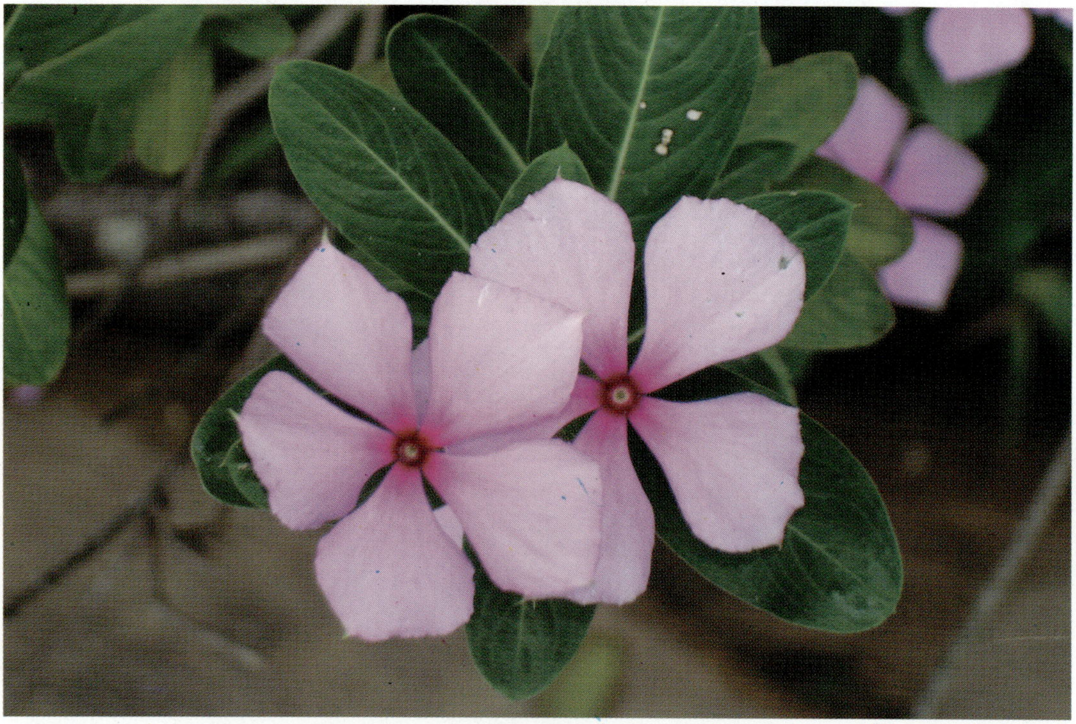

Vinca
Catharanthus roseus

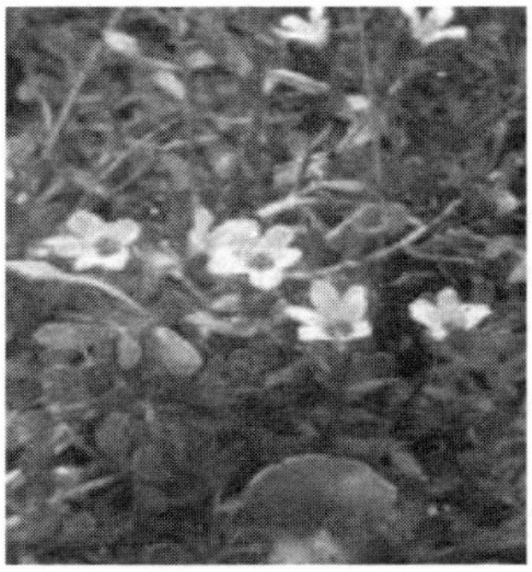

1

Herbal Drug Industry

In This Chapter, You Will Learn

- What are herbal drugs
- Why herbal medicines are gaining popularity
- Growth of the medicinal plant–based industry in recent times
- Status of Indian herbal drug industry and the challenges faced
- Institutions in India that are involved with research in herbal drugs

Since ancient times, human beings have depended on plants as a source for curing ailments, providing long lasting good health, relieving bodily distress and for imparting flavour and aroma to food. A healthcare system centered on plants has been in use in India and China for more than 5000 years. In Europe, plants were being used as mainstream medicines till about 50 years ago. The ancient civilizations of India, China, Greece and Arabic countries independently developed their own indigenous systems of medicine. However, the most superior system in terms of depth of study and coverage is the Ayurvedic system. This system—estimated to have come into being around 6000 BC—is one of the oldest systems of medicine.

In the early twentieth century, when synthetic analgesics and antibiotics were not yet widely available, herbal medicine was the predominant mode of treatment. As synthetic drugs developed by the allopathic system of medicine made rapid progress and promised quicker symptomatic relief, people began to switch over to this system. Today, after a century has elapsed, we have come to realize the limitations of the allopathic system of medicine. Hence, there is renewed interest in herbal medicine. Modern technological advances in Western medicine notwithstanding, many parts of the world—especially the developing countries—continue to rely on traditional systems of medicine for both preventive and curative effects. The World Health Organisation (WHO) estimates this figure to be close to 80%, which is borne out by the fact that most modern pharmacopoeias have at least 25% drugs which are either semi-synthetic or created as prototypes along the lines of compounds derived from plants.

The 1970s campaign by WHO has played a major role in increasing the credibility of herbal medicines. In this campaign, WHO appealed to all the member countries to take concrete steps for preserving their national heritage by promoting ethno-medicine and ethno-pharmacology. It also asked the member countries to step up the use of medicines recognized by their traditional medicinal systems. This has made available significant medical resources to people living in rural areas, who do not have access to modern allopathic medicines.

> *Herbal medicine is defined as a branch of science in which plant-based formulations are used to alleviate diseases. It is also known as botanical medicine or phytomedicine.*

Of late, the term 'phytotherapy' has been introduced as a more accurate synonym for herbal or botanical medicine. The term 'phytopharmacotherapy' has been coined recently to denote the use of herbal medicines in the treatment of diseases. The inclusion of herbal-based products as dietary supplements is yet another recent development. Herbal medicine is fast evolving into a multidisciplinary science—incorporating aspects of ethnopharmacology, toxicology and biochemistry, in addition to botany, pharmacognosy and phytochemistry.

Definition of the term 'Herb'

Botanical definition A herb is a non-woody, seed-producing plant that dies to the ground at the end of the growing season.

Culinary definition Herbs are vegetable products that are used to add flavour or aroma to food.

Medicinal definition Herbs are crude drugs of vegetable origin that are used in the treatment of disease states, often of a chronic nature, or to attain or maintain a condition of improved health.

Phytomedicinals (Plant medicines)

Pharmaceutical preparations like tinctures, fluid extracts and extracts prepared by extracting herbs with various solvents, are called phytomedicinals.

A few botanical products qualify as either food or drugs or both, depending on the specific intent of the user. For example, when used as a flavouring agent in cooking, garlic is a *food*. When it is used to control hypertension, or excessively high cholesterol levels, it is a *drug*. Some people may simultaneously use it for both purposes.

1.1 DIFFERENCES BETWEEN HERBS AND OTHER DRUGS

1. Herbs are *more dilute* than concentrated chemical drugs.
2. Herbs often *contain additional active principles* that may be closely related, both chemically and therapeutically, to the constituent primarily responsible for its effects. For example, digitalis contains about 30 different closely related glycosides, all of which have cardiotonic properties. However, due to small structural variations, they differ in terms of the time required for the onset of action and the duration of the effects.
3. Besides active constituents, herbs often *contain other principles that detract from their specific therapeutic abilities*. For example, cinchona bark has about 25 related alkaloids, but quinine is the only one useful in treating malaria. However, a patient receiving cinchona also takes in quinidine, which is a cardiac depressant, and cinchotannic acid, which is an astringent and induces constipation.

Advantages of herbal drugs

1. They are non-toxic
2. They have almost no reported side effects
3. They are easily available
4. The prices are affordable

About 90% of the medicinal plants used are collected from the wild; of the 800 plus species used by industries, not more than 20 are under commercial cultivation. This process of collecting plants from the wild is a destructive act as it threatens the biodiversity of medicinal plant resources. This in turn can prove harmful to the economy of the country.

The cultivation approach, although more expensive, is more appropriate because it makes the process of standardization easier. Recently, growers have set up cooperative/collaborative ventures that generate income to people of many Asian countries. The spurt in international trade of medicinal plants within North America , South- and East-Asian countries and Europe has a huge impact on the respective economies. Nepal, for instance, is earning an estimated US $8.6 million per year from the export of medicinal plants.

The word 'herbal' has become synonymous with 'green' and this, coupled with the evidence of minimal side effects is responsible for the spurt in popularity of herbal medicines. The demand for herbal medicines by the cosmetic and healthcare industries has grown rapidly in the past few years.

India is one of the few countries that is capable of cultivating most of the important plants used in both traditional and modern medicine because of:

- The availability of vast areas for cultivating medicinal plants
- The wide variations in climate, soil, altitude and latitude that support the growth of different types of medicinal plants
- The presence of rich flora

China and India are two great producers of medicinal plants; they have more than 40% of the global diversity.

It is estimated that the global traditional medicine market is growing at the rate of 7%–15% annually. The reasons for the rapid annual growth rate (about 20%–30%)in the herbal drug market in India are:

- The favourable policies adopted by the Government of India to encourage manufacturers of purely herbal products
- Absence of pricing guidelines
- Patent policy under GATT

According to the National Medicinal Plants Board, Government of India, India has 15 agroclimatic zones and 17000–18000 species of flowering plants. About 6000–7000 of these have medicinal properties that are of use in folk and documented systems of medicine, like Ayurveda, Siddha, Unani and Homoeopathy; 960 species of such medicinal plants are being traded, of which 178 species have an annual consumption level in excess of 100 metric tonnes. The medicinal species are spread over three environmental hotspots in the Western Ghats, Eastern Himalayas and the Andaman and Nicobar islands and India is rightly termed the 'world's herbal garden'.

Medicinal plants are increasingly becoming a major requirement for the food supplement and personal care product industries. Most nutraceutical and cosmeceutical industries are today plant based with promise of enormous economic growth.

The extraordinary increase in the demand for herbal drugs has led to an irrational exploitation of medicinal plants. The resultant scarcity poses a risk to the availability of various valuable plant species. According to Kobayashi, about 16.9 million hectares of forests are being felled every year and converted to agricultural land; this has led to various problems such as short supply, high prices, forced import and substitution or adulteration of crude drugs. The Convention on International Trade in Endangered Species (CITES) of wild fauna and flora regulates international trade of the threatened species. In India, the export of about 56 medicinal plant entities is banned.

1.2 CLASSIFICATION OF MEDICINAL PLANT–BASED INDUSTRY

The various industries dependant on medicinal plants can be classified into 6 categories:

1. Products based on the Indian systems of medicine, such as Ayurveda, Siddha and Unani
2. Over-the-counter, non-prescription products consisting of plant parts, extracts and galenicals
3. Essential oils
4. Phytopharmaceuticals

5. Natural health products including health foods, nutraceuticals and recombinant proteins
6. Cosmetics

Phytopharmaceuticals

Before Independence, the Indian phytopharmaceutical industry was restricted to obtaining quinine from cinchona. Now, the list spans a wide variety of compounds, including morphine, codeine, papaverine, thebaine, colchicine, vinblastine, vincristine, brucine, strychnine, ergot alkaloid, senna glycosides, diosgenin, plant laxatives, podophyllotoxin resin and citral.

Health products

This category includes vitamins, minerals and nutrients or ingredients isolated from plants. These have physiological benefits and reduce the risk of chronic diseases.

Nutraceuticals

This term is an amalgamation of the words 'nutrition' and 'pharmaceutical'. The term nutraceutical is defined as parts of food that have a medical or health benefit, including the prevention and treatment of diseases. It has three constituents:

1. Herbal and related extracts: Anti-oxidants (Vitamins A, C, E, carotenoids and flavonoids) and herbal teas
2. Vitamins and minerals
3. Nutrients

Nutraceuticals also include probiotics, prebiotics, omega-3-fatty acids and dietary fibres.

Probiotics These are living microorganisms that improve the intestinal microbial balance. Example: Bifidobacterium and Lactobacilli species like *L. acidophillus*.

Prebiotics These are substances that reach the colon in intact form without getting depleted by the gastric pH and digestive acids. They selectively promote the growth of colonic probiotic bacteria, i.e., they act as fertilizers for these symbiotic bacteria. Inulin from raw chicory and lactobacilli from sour milk are examples of prebiotics.

Herbal cosmetics

Herbal cosmetics are those beauty products which possess desirable physiological activities such as skin healing, smoothening, and appearance enhancing and conditioning properties.

Categories of herbal cosmetics

1. Products that enhance the appearance of facial skin
2. Hair growth and care products
3. Skin care products, especially for teenagers (acne, pimples)
4. Personal care products like shampoos, soap, powders and perfumery
5. Miscellaneous products

EXAMPLES Aloe vera, amla, almond oil, brahmi, bhringaraj, castor oil, coconut oil, eucalyptus oil, henna, neem, marigold and sandalwood oil.

In India, steps have been taken to improve the quality of Ayurvedic medicines. Good manufacturing practice (GMP) guidelines have been introduced to ensure quality control. Medicinal plant boards have been constituted in every state and by the Central goverment to encourage people, particularly farmers, to take up the cultivation of medicinal plants. Herbal gardens have been developed to create an awareness of the rich heritage of the Indian systems of medicine. Various institutes like NIPER, NBRI, CIMAP and CDRI are playing a key role in defining standards for the Ayurvedic system of medicine.

1.3 CHALLENGES

There are various aspects that Indian manufacturers have to focus on to establish their products in the global markets. One of the most crucial areas is standardization of the entire process involved in the manufacture of herbal products. Right from the analysis of raw materials and in-process testing to analysis of finished products, systems have to be established to stringently monitor every single step in the manufacture. Today, it is not sufficient to test the quality of your product: quality assurance is the need of the hour. This involves designing quality into your product to ensure products consistently meet the prescribed specifications.

To gain validity, herbal products have to pass through the same rigorous testing protocols as their allopathic counterparts which include stability testing, pharmacokinetic profile studies and safety assessment reports. Herbal industries will therefore have to invest in modern R&D, quality control labs and upgrade their documentation techniques to a level on par with international standards.

An integration of modern techniques and traditional knowledge can help the Indian herbal drug industry grow by leaps and bounds and create a reliable brand worldwide.

1.4 FUTURE PLANS

The Kerala State medicinal plant board has undertaken cultivation of medicinal plants over 500 hectares of land to promote cultivation of specific medicinal plants that can meet the raw material requirements of the herbal drug and cosmetics industries. Similarly, with the assistance of the state government and the Centre, the Ayurvedic drug manufacturers in Kerala are setting up a ₹ 62.5 crore company with a hi-tech quality control laboratory and excellent research amenities to facilitate the study of various medicinal plants.

1.5 HERBAL DRUG INDUSTRY IN INDIA

Before independence, India was mainly producing phytopharmaceuticals such as cinchona and opium alkaloids, a few galenicals and tinctures. During the past few decades, the Indian drug industry has undergone major changes. We now have bulk production of plant drugs like digoxin, caffeine, morphine, codeine, papaverine, thebaine, hyoscine, hyoscyamine, atropine, strychnine, brucine, xanthotoxin, sennosides, colchicine, berberine, emetine, quinine, quinidine vinblastine, vincristine, ergot alkaloids, nicotine and pyrethroids.

A number of governmental and non-governmental organizations and institutions in India are presently involved in the scientific study of medicinal plants. Notable among these are the Central Drug Research Institute (CDRI), the Central Institute of Medicinal and Aromatic Plants (CIMAP), the National Botanical Research Institute (NBRI), all in Lucknow, and the Tropical Botanic Garden and Research Institute (TBGRI) at Thiruvananthapuram.

According to Polshettiwar, "In India, there are about 20 well-recognized manufacturers of herbal drugs and 140 medium or small-scale manufacturers. In addition, thousands of *vaidyas* have their own miniature manufacturing facilities. About 1200 licensed small manufacturers in India are on record. The estimated current annual production of herbal drugs is around ₹ 100 crores. This value is low as compared to the production of allopathic pharmaceuticals, which is around ₹ 800 crores. The demand for herbal medicines is increasing and it is estimated that the production of herbal drugs may be around ₹ 4000 crores in the year 2010 AD. There are 1650 herbal formulations in Indian market and number of major plants involved in their formulation is 540." Table 1.1 lists some major players in the Indian herbal drug industry.

A number of plants have been screened for their biological activities. According to an anonymous source, about 3,000 materials from 2,764 plant species have been screened for their pharmacological and chemotherapeutic properties. As a result of this, many new drugs have been introduced in clinical practice and some are in an advanced stage of clinical development. Yet, herbal drugs have not been adopted widely and doubts are raised on the use of herbal drugs for the following reasons:

1. Herbs of different origins are often called by the same popular name.
2. The same plant, when grown in different climatic and seasonal conditions does not have identical chemical constituents or therapeutic effects.
3. The process of collection, extraction, processing and storage of herbal medicines can cause variation in potency and safety.

These factors are responsible for the low acceptance of these medicines in modern treatments. However, all these factors can be overcome by working towards the standardization of herbal drug formulations. This is now becoming important because detailed investigations into the mode of action of herbal drugs have revealed that they are involved in various enzymatic, endocrine and immuno-modulating functions. Several institutions in India are at the forefront of herbal research. A few of these are listed in Table 1.2.

Table 1.1 A few big players in the Indian Ayurvedic drug industry

Name of the company	Examples of products
Himalaya Drug Company	Liv 52, Bonnisan, Koflet, Mentat, Septilin
Dabur Pharmaceuticals	Chyawanprash, Hajmola, PudinHara, Lal Tail
Emami Drugs	Navratan oil, Boroplus, Fast Relief
Baidyanath	Chyawanprash, Surakta, Mahabhringaraj oil
Pankajakasturi Pharmaceuticals	Pankaja Kasturi Breathe EC, Mygrane oil
Cholayil Pharmaceuticals Pvt Ltd	Yakrita, Rumacide-G, Medimix, Cuticura talc
Zandu Pharmaceuticals	Kesari jivan, Triphala guggul, Pancharishta

Table 1.2 Herbal research centres in India

Name	City	Email
CCRAS (Central Council for Research in Ayurveda and Siddha)	New Delhi	ccras_adm@nic.in
NBRI (National Botanical Research Institute) (CSIR)	Lucknow	director@nbri.res.in
National Institute of Ayurveda	Jaipur	nia@raj.nic.in
Interdisciplinary School of Health Sciences	Pune	shs@unipune.ac.in
Banaras Hindu University	Varanasi	vcbhu1@gmail.com, vc_bhu@sify.com
ICMR (Indian Council for Medical Research)	New Delhi	icmrhqds@sansad.nic.in
National Medicinal Plants Board	New Delhi	info-nmpb@nic.in, ceo-nmpb@nic.in
Regional Medical Research Centre (ICMR)	Belgaum	sankhol@yahoo.com
PERD Centre	Ahmedabad	perd@perdcentre.com
CCRUM (Central Council for Research in Unani Medicine)	New Delhi	Shakirjamil@ccrum.net dg@ccrum.net

Table 1.2 Continued....

Name	City	Email
IMPCOPS (Indian Medical Practioners Co-operative Pharmacy & Stores Ltd.)	Chennai	impcops@dataone.in contact@impcops.org
National Institute of Indian Medical	Hyderabad	iihm@ap.nic.in iihm_ccras@yahoo.co.in
Pharmexcil	Hyderabad	info@pharmexcil.com
Chemexcil	Mumbai	info@chemexcil.gov.in chemexcil@vsnl.com
CDRI (Central Drug Research Institute) (CSIR)	Lucknow	director@cdri.res.in
National Bureau of Plant Genetic Resources	New Delhi	director@nbpgr.ernet.in
TBGRI (Tropical Botanical Garden & Research Institute)	Thiruvananthapuram	director_tbgri@rediffmail.com
FRHLT (Foundation for Revitalisation of Local Health Traditions)	Bangalore	root@frlht.ernet.in
ADMA (Ayurvedic Drug Manufacturers Association)	Mumbai	admaindia@vsnl.net

Source Ashok DB Vaidya and Thomas PA Devasagayam, Current Status of Herbal Drugs in India: An Overview, *J. Clin. Biochem. Nutr.*, 2007 July; 41(1): 1–11; available at *http://www.ncbi.nlm.nih.gov/pmc/articles/PMC2274994/*

SUMMARY

- People all over the world use traditional herbal medicines.
- The major advantage of such products is their low toxicity.
- Herbal products are gaining importance in the health care, personal care, nutraceutical and cosmeceutical fields.
- In India, the herbal drug industry is growing at a rapid rate, but in order to sustain the growth, it is essential for Indian manufacturers to insist on standardization processes to establish their products in the global markets.
- Many institutes and industries in India are carrying out research on medicinal plants.

Exercises

Long answers

1. Explain the importance of herbal medicines and the scope of herbal drug industries in India.
2. Discuss the status of the herbal drug industry in India.

Short answers

3. What is the importance of herbal medicines and cosmetics in herbal formulations?
4. Discuss the use of herbal cosmetics in India.
5. Name some institutions involved in herbal research in India and their well-known herbal products.
6. Define (a) herbs and (b) phytomedicinals.
7. Explain the advantages of using herbal medicines.

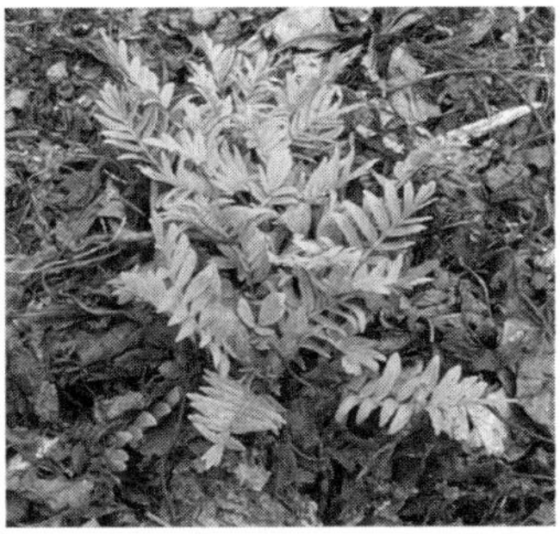

2

Patents

In This Chapter, You Will Learn

- What is intellectual property and what are Intellectual Property Rights
- Definitions of the terms patent, trademark and copyright
- Procedure involved in procuring a patent
- Patents in relation to natural products—what can and cannot be patented
- Plant breeder rights
- Intellectual Property Rights (IPR) in India and the need for vigilance
- Traditional Knowledge Digital Library (TKDL) developed by Indian herbalists

When an individual or an organization invests time, money and efforts in developing something new, making the information public can help further the knowledge in that field. In return for sharing this intellectual property, is an incentive—the exclusive right to that innovation. This protects the contribution from being exploited by others. Like any other property, this right can be mortgaged, sold, given away, licensed, transferred or even just thrown away.

Intellectual property (IP)

The term *Intellectual Property* is used to denote anything that is created by the human mind —literature, art, images, scientific and technological inventions, designs and even names and symbols. There are two classes of IP: one is industrial property and the other is copyright.

Industrial property specifically covers inventions, industrial designs, trademarks and geographic indicators of source.

Copyright includes artistic work, namely, writings, drawings, photographs, poetry, films, musical compositions and architectural designs.

2.1 INTELLECTUAL PROPERTY RIGHT (IPR)

This is defined as the legitimate right of an inventor to protect his intellectual property. This means that others are prohibited from using, copying, making or selling the said property. IPR is a broad term that includes the following:

- *Patent*—for products, equipments and processes with industrial applications.
- *Trademark*—logo, symbol and words that are used to distinguish services or goods.
- *Designs*—appearance or shape that is distinctive to the invention.
- *Copyright*—for any product of a creative process like literature, music and art.

Patent

A patent refers to an exclusive right which is granted to an inventor. The person who has been granted the patent is called the *patentee*. The invention may be a particular product or a process, that is a new method of carrying out an activity or a new way to solve a problem. This right is applicable over a limited duration, which generally is 20 years. If an invention is patented, it implies that no other person can commercially benefit from making, using, selling or distributing it. After the expiry of the patent, however, the invention enters the public domain and can be used by any other person. There is no uniform international guideline for patenting; every country has its own laws governing the process. Some of the well-known patenting authorities include the US Patent Office, the European Patent Office and the African Regional Intellectual Property Organization.

Purpose of a Patent

1. Patents are granted in order to motivate inventors to continue their efforts to develop innovations. This ensures that ultimately, better products and processes are found to improve the quality of human life.
2. Patents give a legal monopoly to the patentee; the patentee can derive monetary benefit from his invention.
3. The patenting system ensures that knowledge is made public. Hence, it is possible for others to do further research on the basis of what is already known. This, in turn, guarantees that there is no duplication of effort and existing systems can be improved at a faster pace.

Procedure for Obtaining a Patent

Although there may be slight differences from one country to another, overall, the procedure begins with the inventor filing an application with the patent office. Details have to be provided in a clear manner in sufficient detail such that even a layman with average knowledge of that field can use the information to reproduce the invention. Generally, diagrams and plans are also attached for easy comprehension. The inventor should also list the claims; this information will decide the limit of protection the patent grants to the invention.

The application is then examined by the patent office for practical usefulness, novelty, non-obviousness and veracity of claims. Most importantly, the subject of the invention should be in keeping with what is deemed patentable by the laws of the country. Medical treatment (not products), plant and animal varieties, mathematical processes, scientific doctrines and natural substances are not considered patentable by many countries. The invention is also compared against a database of previously approved patents in that field. If the patent office sees no reason to reject the application, a time period of about three months is provided for any other party to contest the claims. In the event that no opposition is voiced or the objections are satisfactorily cleared by the applicant, the patent office grants the patent to the inventor.

What can be patented?

Almost all countries have a common set of items that nobody can claim a patent for. The following is an indicative, although not exhaustive, list of such non-patentable items.

1. Mathematical or scientific theory, discovery or method
2. Products of nature
3. Plants and animals other than microorganisms
4. Literary, dramatic, musical or artistic work
5. A method of playing a game, doing some business, presenting information or performing a mental act
6. Some computer programs
7. Methods of various medical diagnosis and treatment
8. Any invention that has implications that go against morality

Patenting natural products

1. Substances that naturally occur as a part of complex mixtures can be patented the first time they are isolated, identified and made available for use. If a process is developed to manufacture such substances for a useful purpose, that can also be patented.
2. In Europe, Japan and the United States, it is possible to patent plants, too. However, the US regulations specify that only plants that are produced by asexual reproductive methods are patentable. The term asexual reproduction refers to propagation methods other than those that use seeds—examples of these include grafting, layering and rooting using plant cuttings.
3. Plants that are genetically transformed (transgenic plants), mutants and hybrids can also be patented. Transgenic varieties like cotton that is herbicide resistant, and an insecticide resistant tobacco plant have been patented.
4. Secondary metabolites produced by cell cultures can be patented. Japan has various patents for the production of the dye shikonin from cell cultures of

Lithospermum erythrorhizon and formation of ajmalicine and catharanthine from *Catharanthus roseus* cell cultures.

5. The term 'plants' includes algae and large fungi, but not bacteria.
6. Animals that have been bred by conventional breeding methods are not patentable.
7. Microorganisms that have been genetically modified to render them significantly different from the naturally occurring species are patentable.
8. Gene patents are readily granted. They typically cover nucleotide sequences, plasmids and other vectors that contain these sequences, organisms that have been transformed by using these sequences and, if it is new, even the protein formed by expression of that particular nucleotide sequence. As per the guidelines of the Human Genome Organisation, patents can be granted only to the complete length of the gene which has some known utility; fragments of cDNA that have no known use are exempt.
9. There are a few natural products that are deemed to be non-patentable. These include plants found to be growing in the wild or those adopted for cultivation, and hybrids of varieties that have been tried for a particular use.

Plant Breeders' Rights

These are certain rights that are conferred upon those who breed a newer plant variety. Also called as Plant Variety Rights, these rights put the breeder in absolute control of all material used in the propagation of this variety, including cuttings, fruits, leaves, flowers, tissue cultures, seeds and divisions. Thus, the farmer who is breeding a particular variety has the right to exclude others from marketing it unless he licenses the variety to them.

In order to qualify for these rights, the variety developed is required to be distinct, new, stable and uniform. Distinct means different from other known varieties in at least one significant botanical aspect like color, height and maturity level. The term 'new' means that the variety has not been commercialized for a period greater than a year. Stability refers to the plant's genetic characters being constant from one generation to another. Uniformity means the characteristics of the plant are the same from one plant to another within that particular variety. The plant breeder who has this right is allowed to give a name to the variety which is then considered its generic name. Anyone who markets this variety has to use this generic name.

IPR in India

As per the Patent Act of 1970, in India, the significant requirements of an invention for patenting are as follows:

- It should be new, that is, not previously present in India or elsewhere.

- It should not have been used in India previously.
- It should be non-obvious with respect to prior art.
- It should be useful.

Further, the Act defines an invention as any new and useful

- art, process, method or manner of manufacture
- machine, apparatus or other article
- substances produced by manufacture, including any new and useful improvements of any of them

In India, the following are non-patentable:

- Discoveries
- Methods of detection, diagnosis or treatment of diseases
- Analytical methods
- Methods of agriculture or cultivation
- Animals, plants and biological methods for rearing and growing them (this does not include microorganisms, though)
- Products like food and medicines made by chemical synthesis

INDIAN TRADITIONAL DRUGS AND PATENTS

In May 1995, the University of Mississippi Medical Center was granted a patent [Patent Number 5,401,504] by the US Patent Office. This was for the use of turmeric in healing wounds. This patent was disputed by an Indian scientist Dr RA Mashelkar—an active crusader for IPR in India. It took four months of hectic activity to prove that turmeric was commonly used in India as a healing agent and antiseptic since centuries. This led to a revoking of that patent.

Shortly after this, in 1996, a patent granted to WR Grace and Company by the European Patent Office at Munich for the fungicidal uses of neem oil was challenged by Vandana Shiva. Drawing heavily from ancient Hindu texts, the European Patent Office was convinced to annul this patent.

However, there are many more such cases where patents have already been granted by the US Patent Office, including traditional drugs like amla, pomegranate, bitter gourd and pepper. These have been granted on the premise that a known compound that is isolated by a known method can still be patented, provided it is intended for a new use. So it happens that pomegranate which is traditionally used for anti-bacterial action has been patented for anti-viral activity. Similarly, pepper that is used for digestive action has been granted a patent for its role in decreasing the dose of Rifamycin.

2.2 TRADITIONAL KNOWLEDGE DIGITAL LIBRARY (TKDL)

Realising the need for vigilance in connection to such patents being filed all over the world, a patent cell has been created in the Indian ministry. In addition to this, the Banaras Hindu

University, Gujarat Ayurvedic University, NIA, Jaipur and Central Council for Research in Ayurveda and Siddha (CCRAS), Delhi, have compiled an indigenously developed digital resource base for preventing patenting of Indian traditionally documented knowledge. This database, known as the Traditional Knowledge Digital Library (TKDL), contains details of more than 2 lakh medical formulations of which 81,000 are Ayurvedic, 1.4 lakh are Unani and 12,000 are Siddha formulations. From the year 2004, over a period of five years, these formulations which were found in Sanskrit, Tamil, Arabic, Hindi, Persian and Urdu texts, were translated into 5 languages commonly used in various international patent offices: English, French, Spanish, German and Japanese. The formulations listed in the TKDL are now designated as 'public property' by the Indian Government: anyone is free to use them, although no one can claim a patent on them or brand them for commercial benefits. This will go a long way to prevent indigenous medicines being patented by foreign companies. According to Randeep Ramesh of *The Gaurdian*, UK, the Indian authorities have found that about 5000 patents for traditional medicines have been issued in global trademark offices, 2000 of which belong to the Indian Ayurveda, Unani and Siddha systems of medicine.

In a landmark treaty that came into force from 2 February, 2009, India has signed a deal with the European Patent Office (EPO), by which it has been agreed that the latter will consult the TKDL before deciding to grant a patent to any company that applies with some innovation based on ancient wisdom. This agreement with a validity period of three years can be renewed repeatedly to continue this vigilance. This agreement also saves the cost of litigation and time. On an average, it takes 5 to 7 years for opposing a patent granted at the international level, which may cost ₹ 1 to 3 crore. Revocation of the neem patent took almost ten years as it involved an appeal case. Recognition and searching from this database at the US, European and Japanese patent offices can guard India against future bio-piracies. For instance, the EPO has already granted 285 patents based on properties of Indian medicinal plants, including papaya, Indian long pepper, hoary basil, mint, ginger, aloe, psyllium, Indian gooseberry, cumin, fenugreek and walnut. As of 2008, there are 65,000 patents on Indian medicinal plants granted by patent offices across the globe.

2.3 PATENTS AND THE INDIAN HERBAL DRUG INDUSTRY

Ever since 2005, when product patents became mandatory under GATT, Indian companies have found the herbal drug–based industry to be a lucrative option. Here, the patent laws have not yet been given a definite structure, leaving greater scope for companies to gain a strong footing. However, one of the leaders in the Indian herbal drugs sector, the Himalaya Drug Company, does not patent its herbal formulations. Applying for patents results in the public disclosure of process details—details that are most crucial for the manufacture of herbal drugs. Although common Ayurvedic texts are the basis for most herbal products, the final efficacy depends to a large extent on the nuanced steps undertaken during the manufacturing process. Himalaya invests a lot in research, testing and validating its herbal products in keeping with internationally accepted standards. It has built up a reputation as one of the leading manufacturers of herbal products. This being the case, it need not rely on a patent to derive economic benefits—keeping its processes secret seems the smarter thing to do.

There is a lot of traditional knowledge lying undiscovered amongst the people living in the interior, and often inaccessible, parts of India. What is needed is the establishment of a network to document this knowledge and also ensure that this information does not get lost with time. Local communities need to be provided some incentives to share this knowledge. A very good example of this is the benefit-sharing model developed by the Tropical Botanical Garden and Research Institute (TBGRI), Thiruvananthapuram, with the Kani tribe that inhabits the Western Ghat region. Based on information provided by the members of this tribe, the TBGRI discovered the anti-fatigue properties of the plant Trychopus sp., which the tribals call Aarogyapaacha. This was later made into the formulation called 'Jeevani'. In order to protect this traditional knowledge and recognize it as the intellectual property of the Kani people, TBGRI filed a patent application with IP India first in 1994 and later, an updated application in 2008. In 2010, the patent was granted, signalling a major victory for the cause of protecting traditional knowledge. Today, the Kani tribals have earned a royalty that runs to lakhs of rupees which is deposited in a trust fund set up for their benefit. What India needs is more such discoveries of the practical applications of traditional medicines that can result in benefits for the true owners of this knowledge.

SUMMARY

- A patent is a set of *exclusive rights* granted by a *state* (national government) to an inventor or his assignee for a *limited period of time* in exchange for public disclosure of an *invention*.
- Trademarks, copyrights and trade secrets are other forms of IPR besides patents.
- There is a global trend towards harmonization of patent laws. The *World Trade Organization* (WTO) is an active partner in this move. The *TRIPs Agreement* has provided a forum for nations to agree on patent laws.
- There is a growing practice of foreign companies patenting medicinal plants and other components of traditional medicine systems.
- A Traditional Knowledge Digital Library (TKDL) has been set up with the help of Banaras Hindu University, Gujarat Ayurvedic University, NIA, Jaipur and CCRAS, Delhi for preventing patenting of documented knowledge.
- India has signed a deal with the European Patent Office (EPO), compelling it to refer to this TKDL before granting patents based on ancient wisdom.
- To prevent patenting of indigenous medicine by foreign companies, the Indian government has made 200,000 traditional medicines 'public property'.

Exercises

Long answers

1. Discuss the relevance of patents with reference to natural products.
2. Discuss how natural products can be patented.
3. Write a note on the current scenario regarding patenting of traditional medicines in India.

Short answers

4. Define the terms IPR and patents.
5. Explain with examples what is patentable with reference to natural products.
6. What is the significance of patents in the herbal drug industry?
7. Discuss plant breeders' rights.

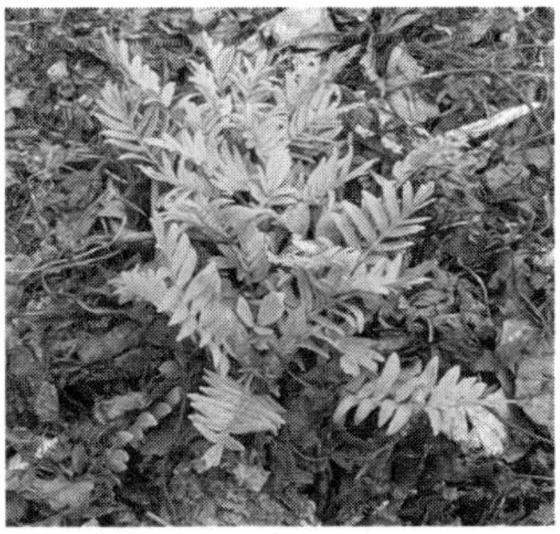

3

Standardization of Herbal Drugs

In This Chapter, You Will Learn

- The various types of plant extracts
- Why standardization is crucial for herbal extracts
- The various components involved in the standardization process
- WHO guidelines for standardization of herbal drugs
- Evaluation of herbal products
- The role of markers in standardization of herbal drug extracts

Although it is generally believed that herbal drugs are safe and non-toxic, it is observed that incidents of adverse effects with herbal products are on the rise. This can be due to various reasons including, but not restricted to, incorrect identification, low quality manufacturing processes and improper labelling.

3.1 DISTINCT NATURE OF HERBAL DRUGS

There are a few properties that are unique to drugs of natural origin; synthetic medicinal compounds are not subject to these issues. A few of these are discussed below.

1. Most herbal drugs are multi-constituent mixtures. Therefore, the activity is often the result of multiple components, many of which may not have been identified.
2. Ever since the modern plant classification system was developed, the botanical identity of many plants has been established. However, many crude drugs unique to certain indigenous systems of medicine, are yet to be scientifically identified.
3. Different collectors may use the same name to refer to two or more plant drugs that differ in their morphological and taxonomical characters. Hence there is difficulty in establishing botanical identity. This is aptly illustrated by the example of Brahmi. Two different plants— *Bacopa monieri* and *Centella asiatica*

have been described as Brahmi. Both have completely different chemical constituents and differ in therapeutic properties. Following intensive scientific examination, the department of Indian Systems of Medicines and Homeopathy (ISM&H) finally proved that the term Brahmi refers to *Bacopa monieri* (called Nira Brahmi), whereas *Centella asiatica* is what ancient texts refer to as Mandukaparni (Brahmamanduki).

Such misunderstandings may not always be innocuous. Adverse effects have been reported with the Chinese herbal drug Fang Ji. The authentic drug called Fang Ji, Han Fang Ji or Fen Fang Ji is the root of *Stephania tetranda*, used traditionally in slimming treatments. This contains the active constituent called tetrandrin. A common adulterant of this drug is Guang Fang Ji, which is so undistinguishable from Han Fang Ji, that even those experienced in handling the two drugs find it difficult to differentiate between the two. Guang Fang Ji is *Aristolochia fangchi*, which contains aristolochic acid—a proven nephrotoxic and carcinogen.

4. Ayurvedic and Unani drugs were in use much before the binomial nomenclature system came into being. During ancient times, many plants belonging to the same genera were often considered as the source of a particular drug. This in itself is not a significant issue. As modern research is proving, drugs belonging to species of the same genus do have similar chemical compositions. However, what is of concern is the fact that the actual concentration of the multiple chemical constituents can vary from one species to another, making it difficult to quantify with certainty the levels of actives in a herbal product.
5. The source of raw material as well as its quality is variable and difficult to control with precision. The various methods used in cultivation, collection, drying, processing and storage vary from one region to another. This coupled with the naturally occurring variations in crop results in a lack of uniformity. Plant drugs are affected by agro-climatic conditions. It is a well-documented fact that the concentrations of chemical components are influenced by conditions like soil properties, level of irrigation, climate, temperature variations, stage of growth and season of harvesting. For example, the leaves of *Adhatoda vasica* show highest alkaloid content during July–October. Hence, harvesting done during any period other than this will imply lower content of alkaloid in the batch of collected drug. Similarly, it is a common practice to dig out *Withania somnifera* roots within 8–10 months of planting, whereas *Tinospora cordifolia* stems are to be collected only when they fully mature.
6. The quality of herbal drugs is also dependent on the appropriate processing and storage conditions. Drugs like Jatamansi roots and *Valeriana wallichi* should be dried at temperatures below 25°C to avoid the loss of major pharmacologically active constituents.

Need for standardization

As the preceding discussion makes apparent, the safe use of herbal drugs is dependent on many factors that are difficult to control. Hence, there has to be a system by which patients are guaranteed a defined minimum level of quality. In other words, there has to be a system of standardization that ensures consistency in quality. This will involve designing quality into each step of the process, right from the cultivation to the final quality control testing of products. Adopting Good Agricultural Practices and Good Field Collection Practices during the cultivation and collection of herbs is a starting step. It is also imperative to develop standard practices to deal with problems in preservation of natural drugs.

Definition of Standardization

Standardization is the establishment of reproducible pharmaceutical quality by comparing a product with established reference substances and by defining the minimum amounts of one or several compounds or groups of compounds.

For herbal drugs, it is very important to develop standardization methods to provide evidence of authenticity, purity and concentration of actives. This term may also refer to the process used to provide extensive quantitative information about the active ingredients present in the product extracts. Among all phytomedicines, the process of standardization is applicable only to extracts.

The standardization process is mainly concerned with adjusting the concentration of herbal drug preparations to a specific content of the active ingredient or ingredients by two methods. In some cases, the herbal extract may be mixed with another batch of the extract of different concentration. In other cases, excipients are used to adjust the concentration of extracts to the prescribed levels.

Benefits of standardization

- Standardization requires a prescribed minimum concentration of active ingredients to be present in the herbal extract. It also stipulates limits for concentrations of unwanted materials that are likely to be present in the extract. Due to this, standardized products are more likely to be of a higher quality than non-standardized products.
- Standardization is a means of ensuring reproducibility of quality.
- Standardized products are necessary in the clinical setting when comparison of products is necessary. The pharmacological effects, side effects and overall clinical efficacy are easy to compare across standardized products. If non-standardized products are used, there is no way to correlate unsatisfactory results with the concentration of actives.
- Products that are standardized provide a greater level of reliability, which gives patients a feeling of security; this also helps in building up compliance.

3.2 TYPES OF EXTRACTS

Several herbal medicines are used in the form of extracts of active ingredients obtained from medicinal plants. These plant extracts are produced by action of a solvent such as water, alcohol, vegetable oils or propylene glycol on the plant part which contains the therapeutically active constituents. The quality of the plant as well as the extraction conditions determines the effectiveness of herbal extracts.

There are three classes of extracts:

1. *(Truly) standardized extracts* These extracts are standardized to active constituents. They are also known as Type A extracts. A typical example is Ginkgo with 26% ginkgo flavones and 6% terpene content.
2. *Quantified extracts* These extracts are standardized to constituents which are known to contribute to the activity. They are also known as Type B extracts.
3. *Other extracts* These extracts are standardized to certain lead compounds. The pharmacological significance of these compounds is not known, but they act as quality markers. They are also called Type C extracts.

Truly standardized extracts

These are extracts where the active constituents are known. The active can be either a single compound or a group of compounds. Hence, they can be standardized to a defined content of the active constituent(s). This, in turn translates into a defined amount of an active in the product. Dry extract of Senna is a good example. It is standardized to 5.5%–8.0% hydroxyanthracene glycosides, calculated as Sennoside B with reference to the dried extract.

In truly standardized extracts, the adjustment of content to a definite value is possible by using inert excipients or by mixing with preparations that possess a higher or lower concentration of active constituents. Such extracts are sometimes also known as *normalized extracts*.

Quantified extracts

These extracts contain chemical constituents, the therapeutic or pharmacological effects of which are known, although the exact group of compounds responsible for the clinical efficacy are unknown. Specialized extracts that contain particular compounds in enhanced quantities are also a part of this category of extracts. Standardization is done by blending various batches of a herbal drug prior to the extraction process. It can also be achieved by mixing different lots of herbal drug preparations. However, concentrations cannot be adjusted using excipients. The extract of aerial parts of St John's wort or *Hypericum perforatum* is an example of a quantified extract.

Other extracts

There are many extracts known to have therapeutic activity. However, there is no information, available on the constituents that are responsible for this activity. It is vital that quality markers are defined for such extracts. These markers provide useful information regarding the quality of herbal medicines and can be a means of monitoring Good Manufacturing Practices. They cannot be used as conclusive proof of the presence of an adequate amount of the active compounds. The aerial parts of Crataegus and *Passiflora incarnate* are examples of this category of extracts.

3.3 GENERAL FLOW OF ACTIVITIES IN STANDARDIZATION

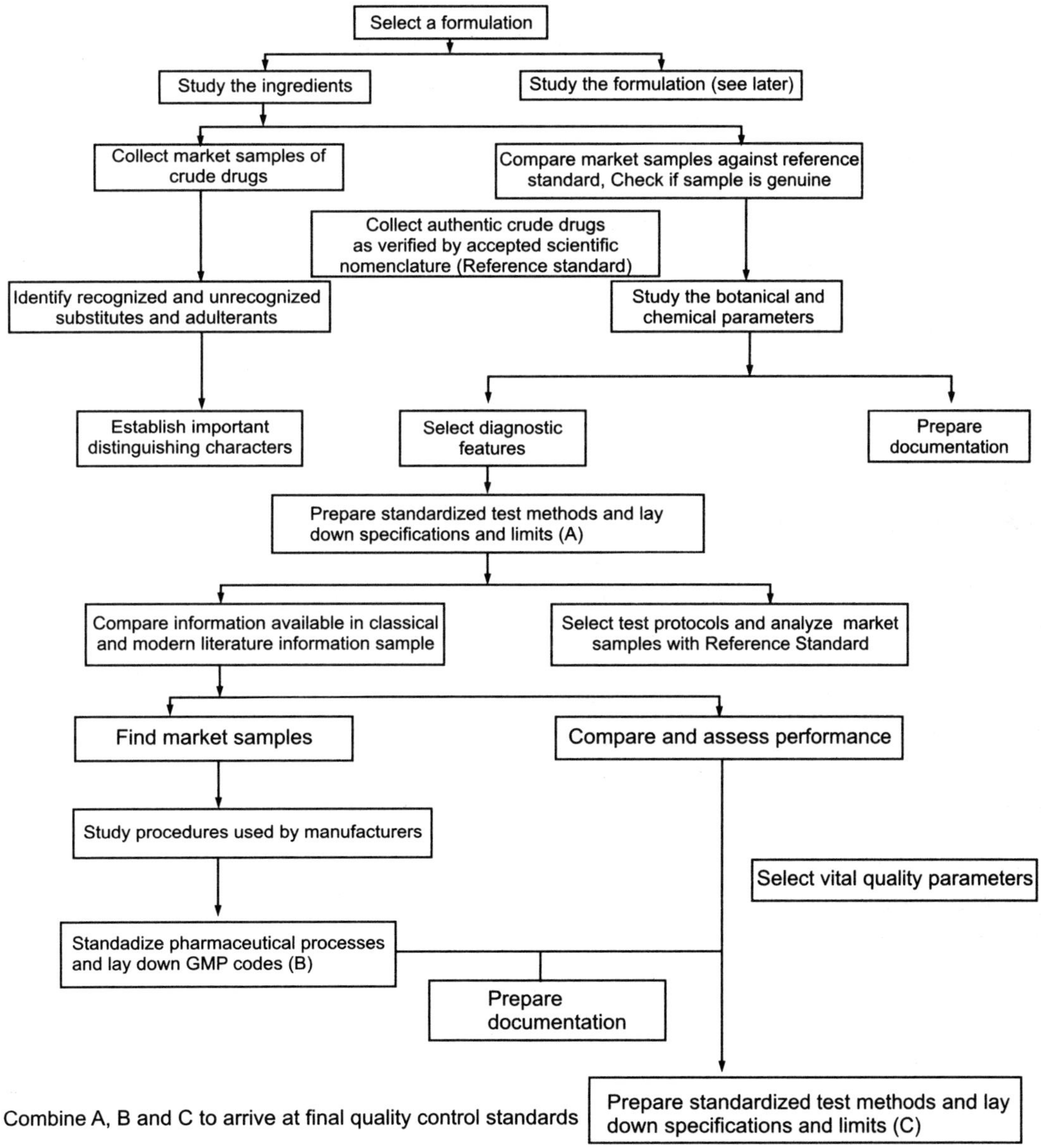

3.4 WORLD HEALTH ORGANIZATION (WHO) GUIDELINES ON STANDARDIZATION

In 1991, WHO prescribed certain standards to be employed in the assessment of herbal medicines. The salient features of these guidelines include the following:

1. Quality control of crude drug material, plant preparations and finished products
2. Stability assessment and shelf-life studies
3. Safety assessment, i.e., documentation of safety based on experience or toxicological studies
4. Assessment of efficacy through the study of ethno-medical information and biological activity evaluation

Parameters

WHO standards for herbal drugs involve botanical, physiochemical, pharmacological and toxicological parameters.

BOTANICAL PARAMETERS (IDENTITY OF DRUG)

- *Sensory evaluation* – visual macroscopy, touch, odour and taste
- *Foreign matter* – foreign plants, animals and minerals
- *Microscopy* – histological observations and measurements

Organoleptic evaluation of drugs

This refers to the evaluation of a drug by colour, odour, size, shape, taste and special features including touch and texture. Observing these traits can give valuable information regarding the identity, purity and quality of the material. This step is therefore of great initial value in comparing a sample specimen with a standard that meets pharmacopoeial quality requirements. This is one of the easiest and fastest methods of establishing the identity and purity and in turn, ensuring quality of a given sample.

Any sample that is significantly different in the prescribed sensory characters like colour, consistency and odour is considered as non-standard.

ADVANTAGE This method of evaluation has the advantage that there is no preliminary treatment required in many cases. In the case of leaves and flowers, it may be necessary to stretch out the wrinkles.

DISADVANTAGE A major disadvantage of this method is that sensory judgment often varies from one person to another. In many cases, it is quite tough to describe the features accurately and characteristics like taste and smell may be labelled as just 'characteristic'.

Determination of foreign matter

Herbal formulations ought to be prepared specifically from the stated plant. They should be devoid of other parts of the same plant or other plants. They are required to be completely free from molds or insects, excreta and visible contaminants like stones, sand, harmful or poisonous foreign matter and chemical residues. Microbial contaminants are another category of possible contaminants of herbal medicines; they are doubly dangerous due to an ability to produce toxins. Macroscopic examination can help in determining the presence of foreign matter. In most cases, microscopic techniques are indispensable in identifying contaminants. In cases where the contaminant is a chemical compound, TLC is the method of choice.

Microscopic evaluation

This is a foolproof method of identifying herbs. It can also help characterize fragments of crude or powdered herbs. This is one of the best ways of detecting the presence of foreign matter and adulterants. A magnifying lens can help to ensure that the plant is the authentic species, and that the drug comprises of the exact botanical plant part. In some cases, however, this may require microscopic analysis. In the case of flowers, for instance, pollen morphology is useful for identifying the species. The presence of particular microscopic structures like stomata is useful in confirming that the correct plant part is used. This is especially significant in cases where various parts of the same plant are intended for use to treat vastly different conditions. *Urtica urens* (Stinging Nettle) is one such example. The roots are used in treatment of benign prostate hyperplasia while the aerial parts are used to treat rheumatism.

Physicochemical parameters

Various physicochemical parameters can prove helpful in characterizing herbal drugs. These include:

- TLC and HPTLC fingerprint
- Ash values—total, acid insoluble, water soluble
- Extractive values—hot water, cold water and ethanol
- Moisture content and volatile matter—loss on drying and azeotropic distillation
- Volatile oils—by steam distillation

Determination of ash values

This is done by burning plant material; the residual ash is measured as total and acid-insoluble ash. Total ash is a measure of the total amount of material left after burning and includes ash derived from the part of the plant itself and acid-insoluble ash. The value obtained after boiling the total ash with dilute hydrochloric acid, and burning the remaining insoluble matter is known as acid-insoluble ash. This value also provides data regarding the amount of silica present in the form of siliceous earth and sand.

Analytical methods

Recent developments in instrumental techniques have simplified the quantitative determination of constituents. More importantly, there has been a significant advancement in the methods of isolation, purification and structure elucidation of naturally occurring metabolites. This has improved the process of developing strategies to analyze the quality of herbal products as well as their standardization.

Analytical methods like thin layer chromatography (TLC), high-performance TLC (HPTLC), quantitative TLC (QTLC), high-performance liquid chromatography (HPLC) and gas chromatography (GC) are useful in assessing homogeneity of plant extracts. Other important tools include over-pressured layer chromatography (OPLC), infrared and UV–VIS spectrometry and mass spectrometry.

Liquid chromatography (LC) used alone, or in combination such as GC/MS and LC/MS and nuclear magnetic resonance (NMR), can also be applied to the standardization and quality control of raw materials as well as finished product. A combined result of the findings of all these sophisticated techniques is helpful in characterizing the chemical nature of impurities present in the herbal product.

Pharmacological parameters

Besides the usual pharmacological testing, a few specific qualities need verification in the case of some herbal products. These include:

- *Bitterness value*—unit equivalent bitterness of standard solution of quinine hydrochloride
- *Haemolytic property*—on ox blood, by comparison with standard reference solution of saponins
- *Astringent property*—tannins that bind to standard Frieberg hide powder
- *Swelling index*—in water
- *Foaming index*—foam height produced by 1g material under specified conditions.

Toxicological parameters

- *Arsenic*—evaluation of the stain produced on mercuric bromide paper
- *Pesticide residues*—including total organic phosphorus and total organic chloride
- *Heavy metals*—presence of lead and cadmium
- *Microbial contamination*—total viable aerobic count of pathogens like Enterobacteriaceae, *E. coli*, Salmonella, *Pseudomonas aeruginosa* and *Staphylococcus aureus*
- *Aflatoxins*—evaluation by TLC using standard aflatoxins (B1, B2, G1 and G2)
- *Radioactive contamination*

Determination of heavy metals

Contamination by toxic heavy metals like lead, copper, cadmium and mercury can be due to various causes that are intentional or accidental. Presence of these heavy metals is potentially dangerous to the health of the person using the herbal formulation. Hence, it is important to limit the proportion of these metals. Pharmacopoeias prescribe the methods used to determine heavy metals based on colour reactions with special reagents such as thioacetamide or diethyldithiocarbamate.

In cases where the metals are present in trace quantities, instrumental methods of analysis are necessary. The methods generally used include atomic absorption spectrophotometry (AAS), inductively coupled plasma (ICP) and neutron activation analysis (NAA).

Determination of microbial contaminants and aflatoxins

- It is common for herbal drugs to contain a number of bacteria and molds, that originate from the soil. Lack of attention during processes like harvesting, cleaning, drying, handling and storage can cause additional contamination with *Escherichia coli* or Salmonella spp. Although a wide range of bacteria and fungi are found, aerobic spore-forming bacteria are predominant contaminants.
- Evaluation of the microbial contamination generally includes determination of the total aerobic microbial count, the total fungal count, and the total Enterobacteriaceae count, together with tests for the presence *of Escherichia coli, Staphylococcus aureus*, Shigella, *Pseudomonas aeruginosa* and Salmonella spp. The *European Pharmacopoeia* also specifies that *E. coli* and Salmonella spp. should be absent from herbal preparations. However, clinical problems are not the prerogative of just these two species; various other organisms are also responsible.
- Materials of vegetable origin show greater levels of microbial contamination than synthetic products. Hence, the requirements for microbial contamination in the *European Pharmacopoeia* permit higher levels of microbial contamination in herbal remedies than in synthetic pharmaceuticals. The contamination level permitted often depends upon the processing the drug has undergone. In herbal formulations that involve boiling with water, for instance, greater contamination levels are permitted.
- Aflatoxins, even in minute quantities, are dangerous contaminants in herbal drugs. They are produced by various species of fungi during storage. WHO prescribes specific procedures for the determination of aflatoxin contamination in herbal drugs.

Determination of pesticide residues

- It is important to have methods of controlling the levels of pesticides and fumigants present in herbal formulations. Most herbal drugs show the presence of pesticide residues. This is due to agricultural processes such as soil treatment during cultivation, spraying of pesticides and using fumigants during storage. It is sufficient to test herbal drugs for the presence of specific groups, rather than for individual pesticides. Most pesticides contain chlorine in the molecule, which can be measured by analyzing the total organic chlorine. Similarly, insecticides containing phosphate can be identified by measuring total organic phosphorus.

- WHO provides details of a few simple procedures; the *European Pharmacopoeia* has general limits to restrict the presence of pesticide residues in medicine. The process of testing includes extracting samples of herbal material by a standard procedure, removing impurities by partition/adsorption, and subsequent measurement of quantities of individual pesticides by GC, MS or GC/MS.

Determination of radioactive contamination

Due to exposure to ionization radiation such as radionuclides, herbal drugs are bound to contain a certain degree of radioactive contaminants. However, dangerous contamination often occurs only in the event of a nuclear accident. WHO, in close cooperation with several other international organizations, has developed guidelines to handle widespread contamination by radionuclides due to major nuclear accidents. The contamination in such cases can have varying levels of significance depending on the specific radionuclide, the level of contamination, and the quantity of the contaminant that is consumed. However, considering the usual quantities of herbal medicines consumed by an individual, radioactive contaminants do not pose a significant health risk. Hence, no limits are currently prescribed for limiting levels of radioactive contamination.

Illustration of Standardization Process

Digitalis purpurea (Foxglove leaves)

The extracts are known to contain glycosides like digitoxin, digoxin and lanatoside C; hence, Foxglove extracts are (truly) standardized extracts.

Quality Control

A. Powder microscopical characters
   - Two-to seven-celled covering trichomes
   - Polygonal epidermal cells and stomata
   - Absence of calcium oxalate and sclerenchyma cells

B. Phytochemical analysis is carried out to quantify active ingredients by HPLC and TLC. However, one of the major problems with digitalis is that cardenolides differ widely in their pharmacological potency. The narrow 'safe dose' range is another concern that necessitates the use of biological methods.

C. Most commonly used biological methods depend on inhibition of the activity of the sodium-potassium ATPase pump. By labelling ATP with radioactive ^{32}P, the resulting amount of free radiolabelled inorganic phosphate is easy to detect.

D. Levels of digitalis glycosides in blood and plasma can be determined by methods like radio immuno assay (RIA) or enzyme-linked immunosorbent assay(ELISA).

E. In vivo biological determination—LD50 in guinea pigs—is estimated by using an infusion of a solution that contains an unknown amount of digitoxin. The survival time of the animals is measured and concentration can be determined by comparing with a standard solution applied to control animals.

Evaluation of herbal extracts

Herbal extracts are prepared by the action of various solvents like water, alcohol, vegetable oils and propylene glycol on the crude drug. The concentrations of the actives in the solvent as well as the actual extraction conditions are important determinants of the final quality of the herbal extract. Water soluble components like amino acids, vitamins and terpenes are best extracted with water, alcohol and propylene glycol, either individually or in combination. Fatty acids and carotenoids can be extracted using oil as the solvent.

All herbal extracts are required to be clear liquids that are free from foreign particles. There should be no evidence of any precipitate or sludge. Prolonged storage should not affect these characteristics in any way.

Colour

Different extracts have different colours, depending on the plant characteristics. Carotenoids from carrot give a red extract while spirulina extracts show a blue colour. A brown-coloured extract may be an indication of improper processing or chemical reactions like oxidation and polymerization of sugar derivatives. It may also signal the start of degradation reactions in the extract.

Odour

Like colour, smell also depends on the nature of the plant. A lack of similarity between the plant and extract with reference to the odour often signals problems with the extract.

Lack of microbial contaminants

Although absolute sterility is not possible, an extract should have not more than 100 non-pathogenic germs per gram. Preservatives may be used to protect extracts from microbial spoilage. However, care should be taken to keep their concentrations low.

Dry residue

The dry residue is contributed by the soluble parts of the plant that have been extracted into the solvent. Greater the starting quantity of raw drug material, greater will be the proportion of dry residue. The chemical composition of the plant decides the values of dry residue. Theoretically, the maximum extractible part of a dried plant is typically around 10%–20%. Estimation of dry residue is done by placing 1 g of the sample in an oven at 118°C for two hours. At the end of this period, a constant mass should be obtained.

Refractive index

The refractive index is dependent on the percentage of residues present in solution.

This is linked to the results obtained on the dry residue test: greater the residue in the solution, higher the refractive index. The nature of the solvent is also a deciding factor.

pH

The pH for most extracts ranges from 5–7 and can be considered as one of the quality indicators.

UV–Visible spectrophotometry

Many active plant constituents absorb UV rays of specific wavelength, which is characteristic for that plant. UV–Visible spectrophotometry is one of the simplest methods offering great reproducibility, and can also help to quantitatively assay preservatives.

Thin layer chromatography

This is a physico-chemical separation method and is sufficient to characterize the extract of the plant.

Densitometry

It measures the optical density of a light-sensitive material; it checks the concentration of active constituents which are spotted on the TLC plates. It can be adapted for both quantitative and qualitative purposes. The only limitation is that results are subject to the quality of chromatographic plates.

HPLC

It helps in the determination of very low concentrations of ingredients at ppm levels. It is used mainly to check the quality of raw materials or their pharmaceutical spray-dried extracts.

3.4 MARKERS

Markers are chemically defined constituents of a herbal drug which are of interest for control purposes, independent of whether they have any therapeutic activity or not. They serve to calculate the quantity of herbal drug or preparation in the finished product if it has been quantitatively determined in the herbal drug or preparation when the starting materials were tested. Ideally, the chemical markers chosen would also be the compounds that are responsible for the botanical's effects in the body.

Markers are pure, single, isolated compounds. They are mostly secondary metabolites with terpene, steroid, alkaloid, flavonoid, aromatic and hetero-aromatic frameworks. They may possess alcohol, carbonyl, olefine, acid, amide and ester functionalities. Marker compounds of ingredients are not necessarily the markers for the formulations.

Some markers undergo transformation and decompose, vanish or generate new markers. Marker compounds specific to multi-herbal formulations need to be isolated. Formation of new markers depends on the various manufacturing processes.

Marker extracts Artichoke (2%–5% cynarin), chamomile (1.2% apigenin/0.5% essential oil), Devil's claw (5% harpogosides), Echinacea (4% echinacosides), Ephedra (6%–8% ephedrine/pseudoephedrine), Feverfew (2.6% parthenolides), ginseng (5%–15% ginsenosides), goldenseal (5% hydrastine), horse chestnut (20% Aescin), *Uva Ursi* (20% Arbutin), Gotu Kola (10% asiaticosides), green tea (20%–50% polyphenols), licorice (12% glycyrrhizin), St John's wort (0.3%–0.5% hypericin), Schisandra (2.6%–4% schisandrins), Valerian (0.8%–1% valerenic acid/ hydroxyl valerenic acid/acetoxy valerenic acid), willow (8% salicin).

Active constituents extracts Ginkgo (24% flavoglycosides, ginkgolides/flavonoids/ bilobalides), milk thistle (80% silymarin), grape seed (95% polyphenols), turmeric (95% curcumin), saw palmetto (90% free fatty acids), green tea (60% catechins), *Cascara sagrada* (20%–30% anthraquinones), bilberry (25% anthocyanosides), pygeum (12% phytosterols), kava (30%–40% kavalactones).

Extracts contain several active principles. Hence, the final effect is the result of a complex interaction between the constituents of the extract and the body. When we use markers, it is possible to calculate the total amount of a herbal drug in an extract in vitro. However, this cannot be considered as an accurate prediction of the behaviour in vivo.

SUMMARY

- Various factors that can affect the actual content of phyto-constituents in herbal extracts include botanical identity of the drug, agro-climatic conditions, methods employed in processing.
- Standardization is crucial for herbal extracts.WHO has laid down certain guidelines for the process of standardization, which involve quality control of the drug at the raw material, in-process and finished product stages.
- The WHO guidelines also emphasize techniques for assessment of safety, stability and shelf-life of herbal drugs.
- Markers are often used in standardization. The marker compound should ideally be the active constituent of the extract.
- In cases where the quality is difficult to assess by using conventional methods of morphology and microscopy, modern techniques like DNA fingerprinting are used to evaluate the quality of herbal drugs.

Exercises

Long answers

1. Describe the importance of standardization in herbal formulations, extracts and raw materials with suitable examples.
2. Describe the WHO guidelines for the quality control of herbal drugs with examples.
3. What are markers? What is their role in the standardization of crude drugs?
4. Describe the parameters assessed in the evaluation of herbal extracts.

Short answers

5. How is HPLC useful in evaluation of herbal formulations?
6. Describe the significance of ash value in evaluating herbal extracts.
7. Write a note on the different types of herbal extracts.
8. Discuss the significance of standardization of crude drugs.

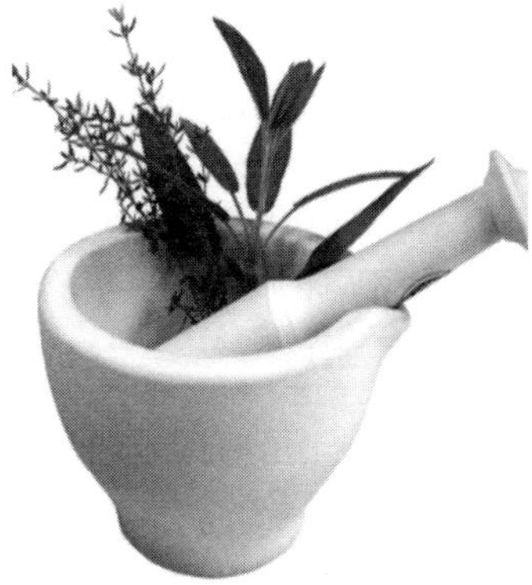

4

Traditional Systems of Medicine

In This Chapter, You Will Learn

- The different traditional systems of medicine
- The basic principles of diagnosis and treatment in Ayurveda, Unani, Siddha, Homeopathy (AYUSH), Aromatherapy and Chinese systems

In recent times, more people are accepting the traditional systems of medicine because of the incidence of uncomfortable and sometimes harmful side effects of the allopathic remedies. There are specific principles in each of these systems for explaining the cause and treatment of diseases and disorders.

4.1 AYURVEDA

The term 'Ayurveda' is a union of the Sanskrit words a*yur* meaning 'life' and *veda* meaning 'knowledge or science'. This system of medicine has been in practice for over 5,000 years. The focus in Ayurveda is not just on the health of the body, but on realizing total health linking the body, mind and soul.

Life (ayu) is the combination (samyoga) of the body, senses, mind and the reincarnating soul. Ayurveda is the most sacred science of life, beneficial to humans both in this world and the world beyond.

Charaka Samhita, Sutrasthana:1.42–43

Around 15,000 BC, Ayurveda had two distinct schools: Atreya, the school of Physicians, and Dhanvantri, the school of Surgeons. Thus, it was a clearly delineated system of medicine. Around 1,000 BC, the sage physicians Charaka and Susrutha wrote the *Charaka Samhita* and *Susruta Samhita,* respectively. The *Charaka Samhita* discusses basic medical sciences like anatomy, physiology and pharmacology. It forms the foundation of Ayurvedic practice. The *Samhita* has been translated into many Indian languages as well as Tibetan and Arabic. The *Charaka Samhita* discusses the pathology of diseases, and their diagnoses; it focusses on the non-surgical modes of treatment using various formulations derived from natural sources. The *Susruta Samhita* discusses prosthetic surgery for replacing limbs, cosmetic surgery, Caesarian operations and even brain surgery. Susruta is famous for his innovative method of cosmetic surgery on the nose (rhinoplasty). Around 500 AD, Vagbhata compiled the third major treatise on Ayurveda, called the *Astanga Hridaya*. This treatise combined information from both the *Samhitas*. Charaka, Susruta and Vagbhata constitute the Trinity or Brihatrayee of Ayurveda. Table 4.1 shows the branches of Ayurveda and their allopathic equivalents.

Table 4.1 Branches of Ayurveda

Branch of Ayurveda	Allopathic equivalent
Kayachikitsa	Internal medicine
Shalakya Tantra	Surgery and treatment of head and neck, ophthalmology and laryngology
Shalya Tantra	Surgery
Agada Tantra	Toxicology
Bhuta Vidya	Psychiatry
Kaumarabhritya	Paediatrics
Rasayana	Science of rejuvenation or anti-aging
Vajikarana	Science of fertility

PANCHAMAHABHUTAS

According to Ayurveda, the whole universe is composed of five basic elements called the Panchamahabhutas, namely earth (prithvi), water (aap), fire (tej), air (vayu) and ether (aakash). Imbalance of doshas leads to ill health. The five elements pervade the tissues and determine the inherent state of the individual (prakriti). It is only when the manifestation of the elements, as dhatus and doshas, is somehow unbalanced, either voluntarily or through external influences, that disease occurs. The growth and development of the body depends on good nutrition. Food, in turn, is composed of the five elements, which replenish or nourish the like elements of the body through the action of the body's fire (Agni).

DOSHAS

The three principal doshas in the body are vata (wind), pitta (bile) and kapha (phlegm). They are found in all living beings. A certain dosha is dominant in an individual depending on his or her inherent state (prakriti). As long as the three doshas remain in the right balance, depending on the prakriti of the individual, there is good health. The perturbation or disturbance of any dosha in relation to the other two leads to disease. Good digestion requires the correct proportion of the three doshas. The normal condition of the bowels indicates a predominance of kapha, while dominance of pitta and vata causes loose bowels and constipation, respectively.

The five elements or bhutas are responsible for the formation of doshas. Vata is created by a combination of earth and air, pitta by a combination of fire and water, and kapha is produced by a synergy of earth and water.

Prana

Prana or life force in our body is said to flow through the seven chakras or psychic energy centres. This energy is described as being of five types—udana, prana, samana, apana and vyana. According to Ayurveda, a blockage in the flow of this energy is responsible for various diseases in human beings. Hence, the treatment procedures correct the imbalance of the various factors.

Ayurveda prescribes the use of specific medicines, suitable diet, exercise and activity, and specific panchakarma procedures to restore the correct flow of energy in the body. This treatment regimen is meant to rejuvenate body mechanisms and restore balance to build health from within, thus minimizing future incidence of disease.

Panchakarma therapy

This is a mode of therapy generally performed in three stages: poorva karma, pradhana karma and paschata karma.

Poorvakarma is the first stage of therapy—preparing the patient, medicines and equipments. These initial procedures are of three types: pachana (digestion therapy), snehana (oleation therapy) and svedana (exudation therapy or induction of sweating)

Pradhana karma is the next stage where the drug is actually administered. This includes various treatments like vamana (emesis), virechana (purgation), vasti (enema), nasya or shirovirechana (nasal insufflation), raktamokshana (removing vitiated blood) or asravisruthi.

Paschata karma refers to the post-treatment procedures aimed at recuperation and consists of diet, medicine and lifestyle changes. It can be of three types: samsarajana karma (specific diet), rasayanadi karma (particular drugs) and shamana prayoga (drugs to treat disease after its elimination).

Ayurveda is at the forefront of medical research as a viable system of medicine because of low potential side effects. Using references from ancient texts, researchers are now trying to isolate the active constituents present in particular herbs to find cures for terminal diseases like cancer and AIDS.

4.2 UNANI TIBB

The Unani system originated in Greece. The Greek philosopher-physician Hippocrates (460–377 BC) laid the scientific foundation for this system, and many other Greek scholars who came after him also contributed to its knowledge base. Galen, Rhazes and Avicenna were some of the scholars who helped develop this system of medicine.

The Arabs introduced Unani to India and the Mughal rulers patronized it. Hakim Ajmal Khan (1868–1927) was an active and scholarly practitioner of this system in the modern era.

Principles

The Unani system, based on the Hippocratic theory, considers the balance of arkhan (elements), akhlat (humor) and mijaz (temperament) as the prime requisites for a healthy mind and body.

The basic principle states that there are four humors in the human body, namely, dum (blood), bhalgam (phlegm), safra (yellow bile) and soada (black bile). There is a specific proportion of all these humors in each individual, responsible for maintaining his or her state of health. The right humoral balance is maintained by an intrinsic power of self-preservation called the *Quwut-e-Modabira*. Any weakening of this power leads to an imbalance in the humoral constitution, which, in turn, leads to disease. Therefore, the treatment in Unani system consists of using substances that ensure that the body regains this power, and balance in humoral constitution is restored.

According to the principles of Unani, there are six essential requirements for the prevention of disease. They are known as the Asbabe-Sita-Zarooriya—air, food and drinks, bodily movements and response, sleep and wakefulness, excretion and retention.

Treatment

The Unani system relies on simple diet control in the initial stages of uncomplicated illnesses, followed by administration of a single drug. If this treatment fails, a compound preparation is prescribed. These treatment systems are known as Ilajbit-tadbeer (regimental therapy), Ilajbit-ghiza (diet therapy), Ilajbit-dawa (pharmacotherapy) and Jarahat (surgery).

Pharmacotherapy involves the use of natural herbal drugs; animal and mineral drugs are also used. Procedures like diaphoresis, venesection, cupping, cauterization, Turkish bath, purging and emesis are a part of regimental therapy. Diet therapy includes the treatment of ailments by regulating the quantity and quality of food or following specific diets.

Diagnosis

A unique characteristic of this system is the manner in which it makes use of the pulse (nabz) to diagnose conditions. Study of the urine (baul) and stools (baraz) are also used in diagnosis of diseases.

4.3 SIDDHA

The word 'Siddha' is derived from the Sanskrit word *Siddhi,* which means a goal or objective to be achieved. Great scholars and doctors with vast knowledge of chemistry and medicine were known as Siddhas or Siddhars in Tamil Nadu and they practiced an ancient system of medicine in India. As per traditional Siddha literature, 18 such Siddhas were revered for their knowledge of medicine and therapy. The Siddha system of medicine relies upon the use of minerals and metals in treating various ailments. Siddha, like Ayurveda, propounds a strong connection between health of the body and the soul. The treatment regimens, therefore, seek to heal both.

Principles

Like Ayurveda, the Siddha system also believes in the system of three humors: vata, pitta and kapha. A balance in these ensures the good health of an individual.

Diagnosis

The physician relies on inputs from eight aspects of the patient's body: general appearance, tongue, voice, eyes, skin, pulse, urine and stools. All the aspects, except the voice, are judged by their colour. Voice is judged on the basis of pitch.

A major feature that distinguishes Siddha from Ayurveda is the emphasis on mineral medicines in the treatment of disorders. Alchemy is a science that deals with converting lower metals into gold or other forms. Siddhars used the principles of alchemy to prepare mineral drugs. The logic behind the use of metals is that the preservation of the body is possible only by using materials that do not undergo decomposition. Another possible reason for the predominance of metals is that these were more readily available than herbs, and hence, physicians preferred to use them.

Medicines used in Siddha are of three classes: thavaram (herbal origin), thathu (metal and mineral origin) and jangamam (animal origin). All these drugs are further classified according to five properties known as suvai (taste), gunam (character), veerya (potency), pirivu (class) and mahimai (action).

4.4 HOMEOPATHY

The word 'Homeopathy' is derived from two Greek words: *homois* meaning 'similar' and *pathos* meaning 'suffering'. Thus, Homeopathy treats diseases with remedies that can produce symptoms similar to the disease when taken by healthy people. The basis of this system of medicine is the natural law of healing called *Similia Similibus Curentur*, which means 'like are cured by likes'.

Dr Samuel Hahnemann (1755–1843) is credited with giving Homeopathy a scientific basis in the early 19th century. During the course of his experiments with cinchona bark, he observed that the effects produced when he ingested the bark were almost similar to those experienced by people suffering from malaria. He concluded that similarity is the basis of healing using herbs, and that only a drug that produces the symptoms in healthy persons can cure the disease in an afflicted individual. By conducting research on a variety of drugs, Hahnemann arrived at the law of similars. The basic principle of Homeopathy is that a vital force in the human body is responsible for the maintenance of health. When a drug is administered, it produces artificial symptoms that activate this vital force to eliminate the original disease symptoms. These artificial symptoms cease when dosing with the drug is stopped.

PRINCIPLES

The basic laws of Homeopathy are discussed below.

Law of similar

It is also called the Law of Cure. This law demonstrates that the selected remedy is able to produce a range of symptoms in a healthy person, similar to that observed in the patient, thus leading to the principle of like cures like.

Law of single remedy

This law directs the practitioner to administer only one remedy at a time. The drug chosen should address the predominant symptom complex of the sick person. Most of the remedies used in Homeopathy have proved active when taken singly. Therefore, a combination of two or more remedies is considered as a new remedy, requiring further research before it can be administered to patients. Besides, this is one of the ways to identify the curative element accurately. Homeopathy also believes that although co-administration of remedies may have a synergistic effect, the probability of adverse effects cannot be ruled out entirely.

Law of minimum dose

The remedy should be administered in small dosage levels to prevent a toxic effect on the body. The principle of dilutions (or 'law of minimum dose') states: the *lower* the dose of the medication, the *greater* its effectiveness. In Homeopathy, there is a step-wise dilution of drugs, with vigorous shaking between dilutions. This process is called 'potentization'. It is believed that this process transfers some of the initial energy from the starting substance to the final diluted form that is administered to the patient. Modern scientists argue against this principle. They contend that the actual concentration of active ingredients in the diluted remedy is so small as to be negligible, and the basis of the cure is questionable. Homeopathic practitioners, however, believe that even the most dilute of remedies retain an imprint of the original drug. This theory, called the 'memory of water', believes that this imprint stimulates the self-healing properties of the body.

PREPARATION OF REMEDIES

The drugs used in homeopathic treatment are called *remedies*. A process of multiple dilutions or potentization, is used to prepare them. Including a greater number of stages of potentization is believed to increase the therapeutic potential of the remedy. Two methods are used to prepare these remedies: multiple vial method and single vial method. The initial solution used for dilution is known as the mother tincture. Compounds that are insoluble are rendered soluble through processes like trituration, grinding and mixing with lactose powder.

Selection of the potency of the product to be administered to the patient depends on factors such as the nature of the disease condition (acute/chronic, physical/emotional), vitality of the patient, degree of confidence the prescriber has on a particular cure and so on. If there are multiple symptoms presented in the patient, the cure proceeds from most important to less important organs, from within the body to outside and from top to bottom. The cure is aimed at causing a removal of symptoms in reverse chronological order of their appearance.

4.5 CHINESE SYSTEM

Traditional Chinese medicine believes in the existence of two elements, Yin and Yang, whose proportions are in a delicate state of balance at any given point of time. Disturbance of this balance is the origin of disease. All body organs contain an element of Yin and Yang, although one organ may be more Yang in its nature, whilst the other more Yin. Hence, this system believes that correcting the imbalance is the key to curing an ailment.

Traditional Chinese medicine believes that the human body is capable of effecting its own cures, provided it is needled or pushed at particular places. This is the theory behind techniques such as acupuncture and acupressure.

This system of medicine proposes the existence of a series of channels that carry and distribute vital energy called as *Chi*, throughout the body. If there is an obstruction to the flow of *Chi* through these channels, it can lead to disease. There can exist occasions when strain can damage the very integrity of the channels. Such diseases are known as *Bi* or pain. Every organ of the body is represented by one specific channel. Therefore, it follows that applying pressure or needles on the acupuncture points on the channel representing a specific organ can cure the disorders related to that organ selectively.

4.6 AROMATHERAPY

Aromatherapy is the use of volatile materials obtained from plant sources. These volatile materials are also called *essential oils* due to the essence they contain. Most of these volatile oils are strongly anti-microbial in action. Recent advances prove their efficacy in the management of pain and nervous symptoms like anxiety and depression. The effects of essential oils are explained by two mechanisms. The first is the actual therapeutic effect of the oil. The second is in terms of the influence that the aroma is found to exert on the limbic system of the brain through the olfactory system. Table 4.2 lists some oils and their action.

Table 4.2 Some essential oils and their action

Action of oil	Examples
Anti-bacterial	Clove, tea tree, cinnamon and rosemary
Anti-viral	Sandalwood, peppermint, ginger and lemongrass
Anti-fungal	Lavender, tea tree, clove and juniper
Anti-inflammatory	Eucalyptus, bay leaf, clove and cinnamon

SUMMARY

- Ayurveda is based on the concept of Panchamahabhutas and Tridoshas, with importance attached to the health of the body, mind and spirit.
- Unani postulates that the balance of Arkhan, Akhlat and Mijaz are the prime requisites for a healthy mind and body. It also believes in the existence of a self-preservative power, which strives to restore any disturbance within the body.
- Siddha, which is popular in Tamil Nadu, is very similar to Ayurveda, except for the stress on mineral drugs.
- Homeopathy is based on the principles of like cures like, single remedies and minimum dosage.
- The traditional Chinese system of medicine is based on the co-existence of two elements called Yin and Yang, which need to be in a state of balance to ensure good health. It makes use of acupuncture and acupressure along with herbs to remove blockages in the flow of energy through channels in the body.
- Aromatherapy makes use of essential oils from plant sources that have specific anti-bacterial, anti-viral, anti-fungal and anti-inflammatory effects. It is also being studied for its influence on the emotional well-being of patients.

Exercises

Long answers

1. Explain the principles of Ayurveda and Siddha systems of medicine.
2. Discuss the principles of Chinese and Unani systems
3. What are the main principles of homeopathy?

Short answers

4. What are the basic principles of Siddha?
5. Explain the different types of treatment in Ayurveda.
6. What is the meaning of Unani Tibb system?
7. What is Chi in Chinese medicine?
8. What are the different branches of Ayurveda?
9. Differentiate between the Ayurveda and Siddha systems of medicine.

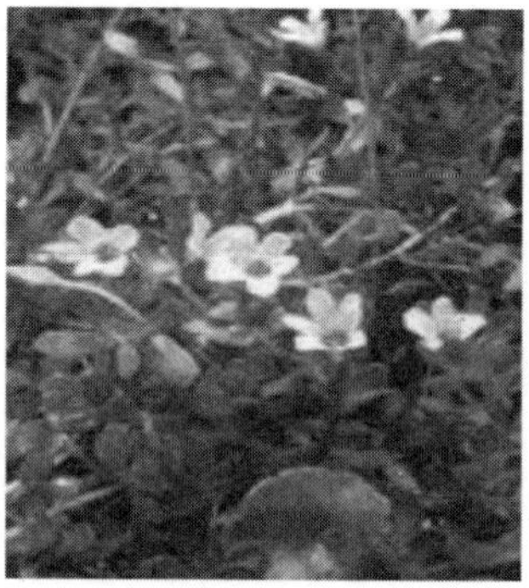

5 Ayurvedic Formulations

In This Chapter, You Will Learn

- The various pharmaceutical processes (samskaras) that a crude drug is subjected to before being used in a formulation
- The different traditional formulations used in Ayurveda such as choorna, asava, arishta, bhasma, avalehya, paka, eye preparations
- The quality parameters used to evaluate different formulations
- Current scenario of Ayurvedic formulations in India
- Examples of commercially available Ayurvedic products for some common disorders

Ayurveda considers the body, the disease and the drug as parts of a whole and not as isolated entities. It appreciates that therapeutic potency is more concentrated in a particular part of the herb. However, it lays emphasis on a concept called *Guna veeryavada* (theory of functional potency). According to this theory, a given herb's usage should be designed to synergize or antagonize the body physiology for the desired benefit. The *Sarangadhara Samhita* is a treatise which exclusively describes the various pharmaceutical processes.

Ayurvedic literature lays great emphasis on the pharmaceutical process termed as *Samskara*, the twin objectives of which are to:

1. Enhance the desirable qualities of the drug being processed
2. Reduce the possible undesirable or harmful effects

Such *Samskara* can be classified into two stages: *shodhana* (purification or detoxification of toxic substances) and *bhaisajya kalpana* (formulation of a dosage form). A number of toxic drugs like *Strychnos nux vomica, Aconitum ferox, Semicarpus anacardium and Commiphora mukul* are purified and rendered safe for use, before they are incorporated into various dosage forms.

Various pharmaceutical processes are prescribed in Ayurveda to achieve the following:

- Isolation of active constituent of the drug

- Easy administration of the drug
- Easy digestion and assimilation
- Better preservation
- Better therapeutic tolerance

5.1 TRADITIONAL DOSAGE FORMS OF AYURVEDIC MEDICINES

The dosage forms depend on the source of the drug and whether it will be used as such or processed further. The methods for refining crude drugs from plants are different from those for compound formulations. These methods are discussed in the following sections.

AUSHADHA KALPANAS OR BHAISAJYA KALPANAS

These methods are used for extracting crude drugs from plants. The resulting extract will be in different forms.These extracts are later used for the preparation of compound formulations.

Swarasa
This yields a fresh extract of crude drugs and has the greatest potency. The whole plant or a part of the plant is plucked fresh. It is cut into pieces, crushed in a mortar and the juice filtered through a thin muslin cloth. Examples of drugs prepared in this manner include ginger (sunti), basil (tulsi) and shaggy buttonweed (vasaka—*Spermacoce hispida*).

Kalka
The fresh drug is ground into a smooth paste in a mortar.

Kashaya or kwaatha
This is an aqueous extract of the crude drug. The fresh or dried drug is crushed and boiled in 16 parts of water and reduced to one-fourth of the actual volume.

Hima or shweta kashaya
This is a process of extracting cold decoction. One part of the crushed drug is soaked overnight with six parts of water in an earthen pot. This is then filtered and used. It can be used for a single drug or two or more drugs in combination.

Phaanta or Faanta (hot infusion)
This is a process of hot infusion. One part of the crushed drug is placed in 4 or 8 parts of freshly boiled water for 12 hours, filtered and used.

Compound formulations

The following methods are used for compound formulations. The preparations use some products from bhaisajya kalpana and subject them to further processing to obtain the formulations. One has to be careful about the exact method of preparing the various formulations.

Choornam

It is a dry or fine powder that can be ingested or used topically. The powder mixtures are prepared by pounding dry minerals, animal or vegetable matter with a pestle in a mortar. Increasing fineness of the powder improves therapeutic efficacy of the drug. In the preparation of compound choornas, each drug is powdered separately and then mixed. The powder is passed through cloth, linen, or a fine sieve, and finally through an 80-mesh sieve.

Choornas may be administered by mixing with ghee, oil, honey, hot water or milk. If jaggery is used, it should be in a proportion equal to that of the choorna. If sugar is used the quantity should be double that of the choorna. Asafoetida, if used, should be baked over fire before adding it to the choorna, since this prevents nausea. Choorna prepared without mechnanical aids is considered more effective.

Choornas are often administered in the later stages of several maladies, and need to be given in bulk doses. They have quick but temporary action. The efficacy of a choorna depends on the time of administration in relation to the disease, hour of the day, before or after meals and so on. Of all the Ayurvedic formulations, choornas have the mildest action and therefore, are less likely to cause unpleasant or toxic effects..

Examples Pippali choornam, ashwagandha choornam, rasanadi choornam, sudarshana choornam and narayana choornam.

Arishtas and asavas

These are medicinal preparations prepared by fermentation and contain alcohol. The powder or decoction is mixed with sugar or jaggery and left for a given duration (7–10 days in summer and 15–30 days in winter). The alcohol generated during fermentation facilitates extraction of the active principles of the drug. It also acts as a preservative.

An asava is obtained from fermented raw vegetable juices, while an arishta is obtained by fermenting the decoction of a drug.

Arishta

A kashaya is first prepared from the crude drug. It is then filtered and transferred to an earthen pot. Sugar or jaggery is added and the mixture is boiled until the ingredients are completely dissolved. (Note:When honey is used, the mixture should not be boiled.) The mouth of the pot is then covered with an earthen lid, sealed with a clay-smeared cloth wound in seven concentric layers. This pot is kept in a temperature-controlled room or on a heap of paddy to maintain constant temperature. After fermentation, the liquid is decanted, strained and bottled.

Some common arishtas are dashamoolarishta, balarishta and jeera arishta.

Asavas

Only new earthen vessels should be used for the preparation of asavas. Water should be boiled first in these vessels before using them for the preparation of asavas. The interior of these vessels should be smeared or fumigated with pepper (*Piper longum*) powder; ghee should also be smeared before use. Sugar syrup is prepared by boiling the mixture of the specified quantity of sugar or jaggery and water. This syrup is cooled and poured into the earthen pot, which has been smeared with a decoction of the drug. The earthen vessel is then covered with a lid, sealed by a clay-smeared cloth wound in seven concentric layers. This container is left to ferment in an underground cellar for about a month.

Some important asavas are kumari asava, madhuk asava and chandan asava.

The quality parameters for asavas and arishtas are as follows:

1. The liquid should be clear without any foam at the top.
2. The liquid should not be sour.
3. The preparation should have the characteristic aromatic and alcoholic odour.

Arkas (Araks or Arkams)

These are distilled essences made by soaking the drug in water for 24–48 hours and then extracting their essence by distillation. These products are usually equivalent to the aqua or 'waters' of the British *Pharmacopoeia*. They are used in fever, dyspepsia and topically as cooling lotions. They mainly contain the volatile oils present in the drug.

Some common arkas are ajamod araka, karpooradhi araka and jatamansi araka.

Avalehya, Leha and Paaka

These are linctuses, confections or thickened extracts. They are semisolid preparation of drugs prepared by boiling sugar, jaggery or sugar candy with the prescribed drug powder or decoction. The jaggery or sugar candy is dissolved in water, boiled and strained. The powdered drug is added in small quantities and stirred continuously to form a homogenous mass. Ghee or oil should be added when the preparation is hot, whereas honey should be added only when cooled. If jaggery is used, the proportion is twice the quantity of the drug, while it is four times for sugar, water, milk or cow's urine. These products are generally used for digestive and respiratory problems, and for general tonic effect on the body.

Some examples are chyawanprash, punarnavaadi lehya and agastya rasayana.

The quality parameters for an avalehyas are as follows:

- It should sink in water without spreading.

- It should not readily dissolve in water.
- It should be capable of being drawn out in threads or wires.
- It should emit a sweet smell.
- In preparations with ghee or oil, it should be possible to roll it between fingers.

Bhasmas

Bhasma means the powder of a compound (metals, minerals or animal products) obtained after purification and calcination. They are grey, whitish, yellowish or black powders. They are quite stable and maintain their potency over a long time. They are easily assimilated and directly accelerate the metabolism. They have a definite action on the endocrine glands. Bhasmas should always be stored in glass-stoppered bottles.

Bhasmas have the following properties:

- A bhasma is not fit for internal administration unless it is nirustha, i.e., it forms a stable compound with the reagent. If not, the preparation may dissociate to re-form the original metal and this may lead to untoward symptoms.
- All bhasmas have a common earthy taste; the colour, however, varies with the method of preparation.
- The older the preparation, the greater is the efficacy and safety of the remedy.
- Bhasmas show minor variation in therapeutic action, depending on the vehicle of administration and the stage of the disease.

The preparation of a bhasma includes two steps: purification (shodhana) and calcination (maarana).

Purification or shodhana

It is done to remove harmful matter, convert some characteristic of the drug, enhance therapeutic action and potentiate the drug.

There are two types of shodhana:

- saamanya shodhana or dipping in oil or cow's urine (gomutra)
- vishesha shodhana, which involves one of the following methods.

Bhaavana	grinding with special drug decoctions
Swedhana	converting the drug into a poultice.
Nirvaapana	incinerating to red-hot and dipping into liquids like swarasa, oil, thaila, etc.
Mardana	rubbing or triturating with some dravyas to remove impurities.

Calcination

The metal or mineral obtained after the process of purification is ground or triturated with the drug decoction and small drug cakes are prepared. These are filled into shallow earthen vessels and closed with a lid. The edges are sealed with a clay-smeared cloth wound in seven concentric layers. A pit is dug in the ground and cow dung cakes with depressions in the middle to hold the vessels are placed inside. The sealed vessels are then lowered into the pit. A fire (puta) is ignited from all sides for complete incineration. Following this, the vessels are cooled, the seal is broken and the contents are removed. The incinerated product is again triturated with drug juice or decoction and the puta process is repeated again. The final dried ground product is the bhasma.

Some examples are tamara bhasma, swarna bhasma, shankha bhasma and loha bhasma.

A bhasma powder that floats on water is of the best quality.

Kshara

These are alkaline substances obtained from the ash of crude drugs. The drug is ground to a coarse powder. An earthen pot containing the powder is heated over fire until the drug inside turns to ash. The pot is then allowed to cool and water is added. The mixture is stirred well and strained through a piece of cotton cloth. The clear liquid obtained is heated over medium fire until all the water evaporates. The salty solid substance left in the vessel is called kshara. Sometimes this may be mixed with other bases like honey, ghee, oil or milk.

Some important ksharas are apamarga kshara and khadari kshara.

Gutikas or gulikas

Gutikas are large pills, tablets or boluses. The decoction of vegetable substances is reduced to a thick consistency and then some powders of drugs are added. Substances like water, raw sugar, honey, gums or gugguls are added to increase the mass of the pill. These pills are intended to be swallowed whole with water, or chewed with honey.

Gutikas are milder than bhasmas and rasanayanas, but are less durable and deteriorate when exposed to air. They should be kept away from moisture if they contain salt, kshara or sugar. The advantage of these pills is that they can be easily administered to children, the elderly and pregnant women.

Examples of gutikas are gandhakavadi gutika, lasunadi gutika and vilvadi gutika.

Gutikas of good quality should not lose their original colour, odour, taste or form on standing.

Thailam or thailas

These are medicated oils and are also called sneha kalpa or paaka. They are prepared by cooking the juice, decoction or the paste of drugs with oil. Unless otherwise specified, the proportion of paste of the drug should be one-fourth while the liquid (drava) should be four times that of the oil. That is, the ratio of vegetable drugs in paste form to oil and water should be 1:4:16. If no liquid is specified in the recipe, water should be used. Usually thailams are internally administered with warm water or milk. These products retain their potency for about 16 months.

The base called sneha is usually coconut oil, gingelly oil or ghee. This is boiled with the kalka or kashaya. When the thaila is completely cooked, a lot of foam appears at the top. This foam should be strained and removed before packing. Any salt or alkali in the recipe should be added after straining. This preparation is called ghritapaakam.

There are three types of ghritapaakams depending on their intended use:

Mrudu paakam	It is a waxy mass which is used in major preparations.
Madhyama paakam	It is harder and used internally or for enemas.
Kharapaakam	It has a sand-like consistency and is used in preparations for external use.

Method of preparation

Thailams can be prepared by two methods:

- The drug is mixed with water or milk and boiled. Oil is then added and the product is heated until the water evaporates.
- Turmeric powder is then added to purify it. The oil is then taken in an earthen, copper or iron pan and gently heated while adding the kalka or fluids. This mixture is then boiled until the water evaporates and the oil is free from froth. The resulting preparation is then strained through muslin cloth.

Some important examples of thailas are vishnu thaila, bhringaraja thaila, jyotismati thaila and prasaran thaila.

Thailas should have the following characteristics:

- It should have a bright colour.
- It should have the odour and taste of the crude drugs that have been added.
- It should have a good spreading consistency.

GHRUTAPAAKA These preparations are similar to thailas except that the final product is boiled until the froth escapes fully. These ghrutas have a dark colour and solidify when cooled.

Some examples are lalyan ghrutam and ashtanga ghrutam.

YAMAKA SNEHA Here the base is oil, ghruta or vasa, which is the fatty oil extracted from flesh (maamsa) or bone marrow (majja).

Pishti

This is a type of bhasma prepared by omitting the process of calcination. After purification, the solid is mixed and triturated with the drug decoction and then dried in the sun or by moonlight.

Mukta pishti and manikya pishti are examples of pishti.

ANJANA, VARTHI AND NETHRABINDU

These are common eye preparations.

Anjana A semisolid preparation of drug decoction is made in camphor. Honey is often added as a diluent or solvent. Nalikena anjana is an example.

Varthi A semisolid mass of the drug is dried and rolled into small sticks. These are made into a paste with honey or rose water at the time of use.

Nethra bindu These are eye drops containing the drug decoction in coconut oil or honey.

LEPANA OR LEPAA

These are used only for external applications. The drug powder is mixed with water, cow's urine, oil or ghee to form a smooth paste.

Kumkumadi lepam is an example.

PAANAKAM

Here sugar syrup is mixed with a decoction of the drug until it attains a syrupy consistency.

Saaribaadi paanakam, aravinda paanakam, panchatikta paanakam and jambeeraadi paanakam are a few examples.

5.2 CURRENT SCENARIO OF AYURVEDIC FORMULATIONS IN INDIA

Commercial production of Ayurvedic medicines commenced about 150 years ago. Prior to this, vaidyas used to collect raw materials and process the required formulations in small quantities. During the Indian independence movement, emphasis on Ayurvedic medicines was revived with a view to inculcate patriotism. In order to meet the growing demand, commercial production began. This has led to many positive and negative consequences.

Advantages

- *Global reach for products* Mass production of Ayurvedic products has led to their widespread availability. Drugs from flora and fauna limited to certain geo-climatic zones can be delivered globally.
- *Professional pharmaceutics* Because of large-scale production, the vaidya could be relieved of *bhaishajya kalpana* (pharmaceutics). As a result, he could concentrate on diagnosis and treatment.
- *Creative marketing strategies* Because of dynamic marketing approaches, certain Ayurvedic medicines have become a household name. The promotion and popularization of Ayurvedic products has resulted in greater interest in the system as a whole.
- *Scope for research and development* Due to the growing competition, the industry has opted to invest in research and development of new products and processes. This has greatly improved the quality and potential of Ayurvedic medicines.

Disadvantages

- *Lack of standardization* Many of the processes described in ancient literature are not designed for production on an industrial scale. Due to a lack of standardization parameters, the initial phase of transition was tough.
- *Pressure on raw material resources* The spurt in demand has placed greater pressure on the raw material resources. This has led to environmental degradation, extinction and loss of biological 'sinks'. It has also resulted in sub-standard materials being used as inputs.

Some common Ayurvedic medicines used for chronic degenerative diseases are listed in Table 5.1.

Table 5.1 Ayurvedic medicines for some chronic degenerative diseases

Name of the disease	Name of the Medicine/ Manufactures	Prime ingredient(s)
Arthritis	Mahayograj Guggulu (Dabur)	*Commiphora mukul*
	Rheumayog (Zandu)	Swarna Bhasma
	Lavanbhaskar Churna (Dabur)	Edible salts and *Punica granatum*
Common digestive problems: indigestion, flatulence etc.	Hingwashtak churna (Dabur)	*Ferula narthex*
	Gufizyme (Gufic)	Calcined copper
	Jeerakadyrishata	*Cuminum cymimum*
Hyperacidity	Zulcer (Nukem)	*Emblica officinalis*
Peptic ulcers	Adliv (Albert David)	*Curcuma longa, Berberis aristata*
	Avipattikar churna	Triphala
Hepatoprotective	Jaundex (Sandu)	*Andrographis paniculata*
	Brahmi vati	*Picrorrhiza kurroa*
	Saraswata ghrit	*Bacopa monierri*
Anti-stress, adaptogentic/ Memory enhancers	Stresscom (Dabur)	*Acorus calamus*
	Mentat (Himalaya)	*Withania somnifera*
	Bravobol (BAN)	*Withania somnifera*
Anti-oxidants	Chyawanprash Awaleha (Dabur)	*Hydrocotyle asiatica*
	Amritkalash (Maharichi)	*Emblica officinalis*
Diabetes Mellitus (non-insulin dependant)	Yasada Bhasma	*Terminalia chebula*
	Nyagrodhadi churna	*Pterocarpus marsupium*
	Madhulene (Trigunayu)	*Gymnema sylvestre*
General skin diseases	Kaishora guggulu	*Euphorbia nerifolia*
	Greneem (Dabur)	*Azadirachta indica*
	Surakta (Baidyanath)	*Rubia cordifolia*
Wound healing	Jatyadi tail	*Curcuma longa*
	Cutfar (BAN)	*Jasminum officinale*
Heart diseases	Arjunaristhta	*Terminalia arjuna*
	Arjin (Alarsin)	*Baliospermum montanum*
	Prabodh (Trigunayu)	*Terminalia arjuna*
Urinary stones	Gokshuradi guggulu	*Tribulus terrestris*
Urinary tract diseases	Stonone (Yogi)	*Boerhaavia diffusa*
	Bangshil (Alarsin)	*Butea frondosa*

SUMMARY

- Ayurveda makes use of several pharmaceutical processes called samskaras to enhance the desirable qualities of the drug and to reduce the possible undesirable or harmful effects.
- The major types of Ayurvedic formulations are choorna, arishta, asava, bhasma and paaka. Each of these has specific methods of preparation and quality parameters to judge the final product.
- Materials like honey, sugar, jaggery, milk and cow's urine have an important role in most of the preparations.
- With the onset of commercial production of Ayurvedic medicines that adhere to quality standards, there is a revival of interest in this ancient mode of treatment.

Exercises

Long answers

1. How are choorna and leha prepared?
2. Describe the basic principles involved in the production of bhasma.
3. Discuss the principles and methods of production of gutikas.
4. Write short notes on: (i) Arishta and (ii) Lehya.
5. Discuss the principles and methods of production of asava and arishta.

Short answers

6. List the different traditional formulations of Ayurveda.
7. What are the merits and demerits of Ayurvedic formulations?
8. Describe the methods of preparation of thaila.
9. Distinguish between asava and arishta.

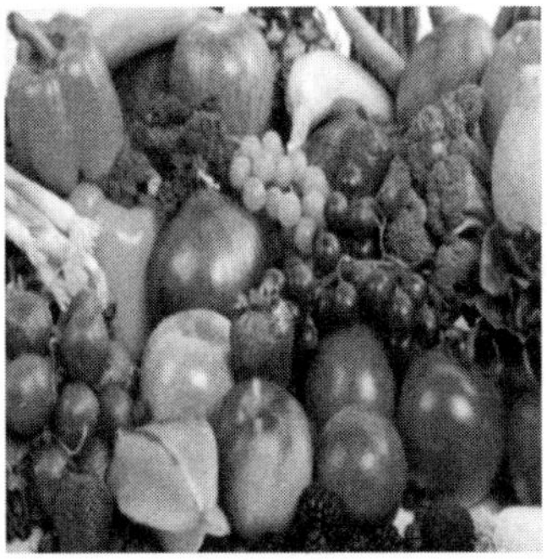

6

Traditional Drugs

In This Chapter, You Will Learn

- The drugs that have been used for many years in traditional Indian systems of medicine
- The biological source, family, morphological characteristics, chemical constituents and uses of some traditional drugs

Since ancient times, plants have been used to relieve pain and cure ailments. The active constituents present in plants affect the human body in different ways. More than one hundred chemicals derived from plants are being used around the world. Some of these substances are listed in Table 6.1. Many of the commercially available drugs are simple synthetic modifications or copies of naturally obtained substances.

Table 6.1 Plant sources, active constituents and clinical action of some drugs

Drug/Chemical	Action/Clinical use	Plant source
Ajmalicine	Circulatory disorders	*Rauwolffia sepentina*
Andrographolide	Bacillary dysentery	*Andrographis Paniculata*
Bromelain	Anti-inflammatory, proteolytic	*Ananas comosus*
Colchicine	Anti-tumour agent,gout	*Colchicum autumnale*
Digitoxin	Cardiotonic	*Digitalis purpurea*
Physostigmine	Cholinesterase inhibitor	*Physostigma venenosum*
Quinidine	Anti-arrhythmic	*Cinchona ledgeriana*
Scopolamine	Sedative	*Datura speciel*
Vinblastine	Anti-tumour, anti-leukemic agent	*Catharanthus roseus*

This chapter discusses some of the traditional drugs used commonly in herbal medicine in India. These drugs are presently being explored for their ability to treat a wide variety of medical conditions; especially those in which the allopathic system is either insufficient or disadvantageous.

6.1 SATAVARI

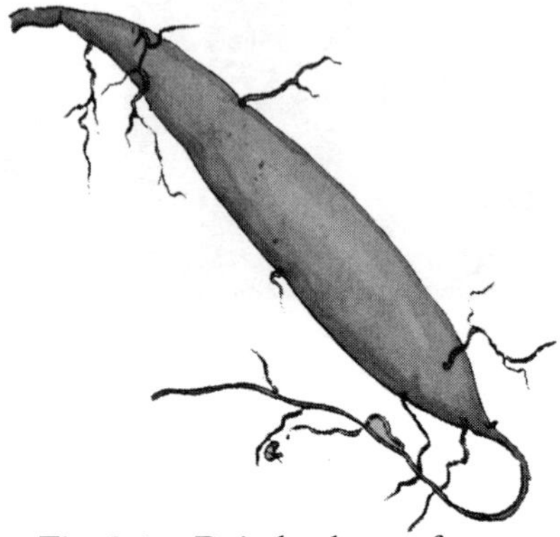

Fig 6.1 Dried tubers of satavari

Common name : Shakakul, Chatwal, Satawar (from Hindi)

Biological source : Dried tuberous roots of *Asparagus racemosus*

Family : Liliaceae

Morphology

Plant : Climber, 1–2 m long
Leaves : Shiny, small, green, uniform, pine-like needles
Flowers : White and tiny with small spikes
Roots : Grey, adventitious, clustered, finger-like, tuberous, tapering at both ends, swollen at the centre
Fruits : Globose, pulpy berries, purplish black when ripe
Surface : Smooth in fresh samples and longitudinally wrinkled in dried ones
Fracture : Complete

Chemical constituents: Contains steroidal glycosides, bitter glycosides, asparagins and flavonoids. The plant contains four saponins — Shatavarin I–IV. Shatavarin IV is a glycoside of Sarsasapogenin with two molecules of rhamnose and a single molecule of glucose. Mucilage and starch are also present.

Uses

- It is used as a tonic and rejuvenative.
- It has anti-oxytocic and anti-abortifacient properties and helps in the shrinking of the uterus after delivery.
- It is a galactogogue, diuretic and anti-dysenteric.
- It has anti-cancer properties and is a good adaptogen.
- It helps in boosting immunity.
- In combination with Ashwagandha, it has been found to hasten the healing of fractures.

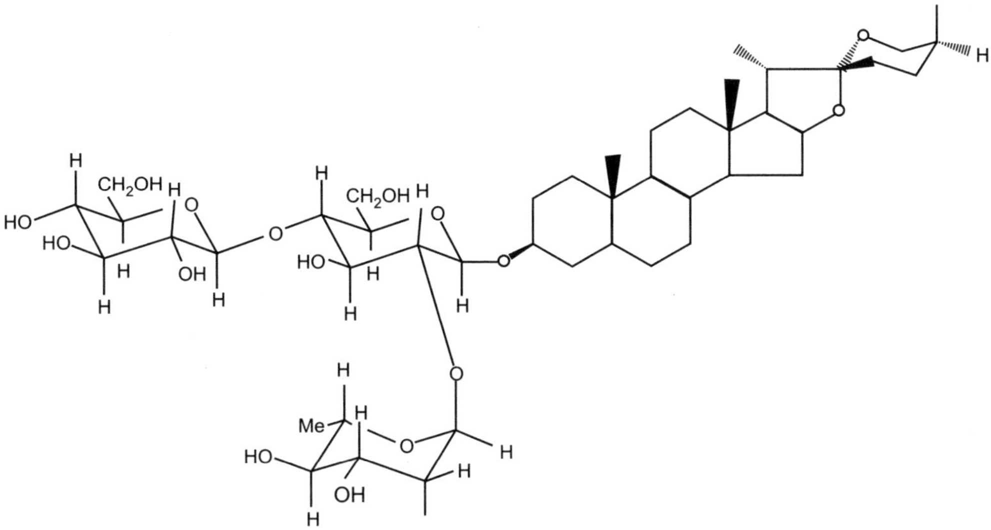

3-0-[a-L-rhamnopyranosyl-(1→ 2) β-D-glucopyranosyl (1→ 4)-0-β-D-glucopyranosyl]-25(S)-spirostan-3β-ol

Shatavarin IV

6.2 KANTAKARI

Common name : Kateli
Biological source : Dried ripe fruits of *Solanum xanthocarpum*
Family : Solanaceae
Morphology
Plant : Prickly, perennial, branched; branches bear dense star-shaped hair
Leaves : Egg-shaped, prickly, sparsely hairy
Flowers : Purple
Fruits : White or yellow coloured, globular drooping and loamy
Seeds : Small, reniform, yellow-brown colour, bitter tasting

Chemical constituents: Steroidal alkaloids such as solasodine and solanin; sterols such as cholesterol and derivatives of phytosterol.

Uses

- It increases micturition and is hence used in the treatment of dropsy.
- It is a steroidal precursor and has aphrodisiac effects.
- It is used in the treatment of sore throat and tonsillitis.
- The roots are used to treat snake and scorpion bites.

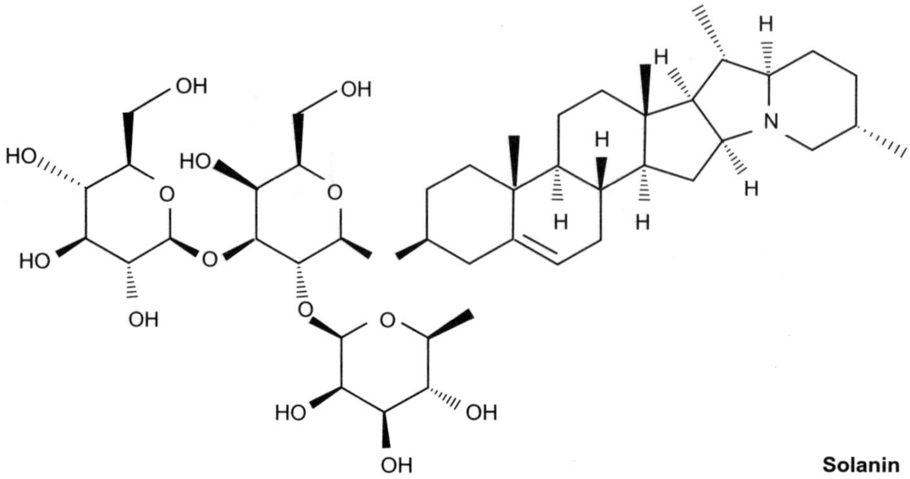

Solanin

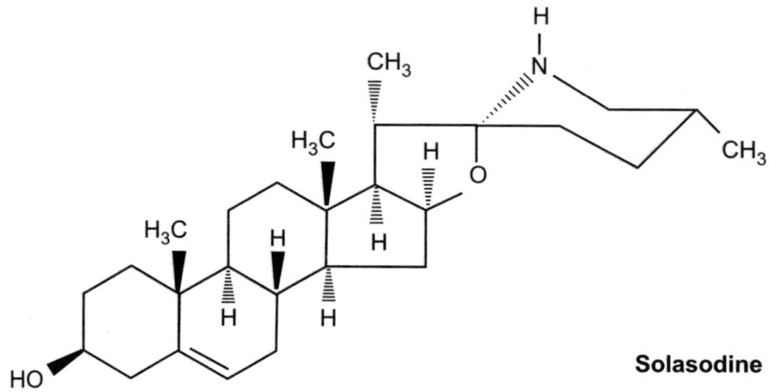

Solasodine

6.3 BAEL

Common name : *Bilva, Shriphal*
Biological source : Whole unripe or half ripe fruits of *Aegle marmelos*
Family : Rutaceae
Morphology

Plant : 18 m long, with thorns and fragrant flowers.
Fruits : Sub-globose berry, with a hard, woody skin. Ripe fruits are yellow-brown, raw ones are green, 7–20 cm in size.
Seeds : Numerous, covered with fibrous hair, set within a thick, aromatic pulp.

Chemical constituents: Coumarins like marmesin, imperatorin, alloimperatorin, xanthotoxol, scoparone, scopoletin, umbelliferone, psoralen, marmelide, tannins and reducing sugars

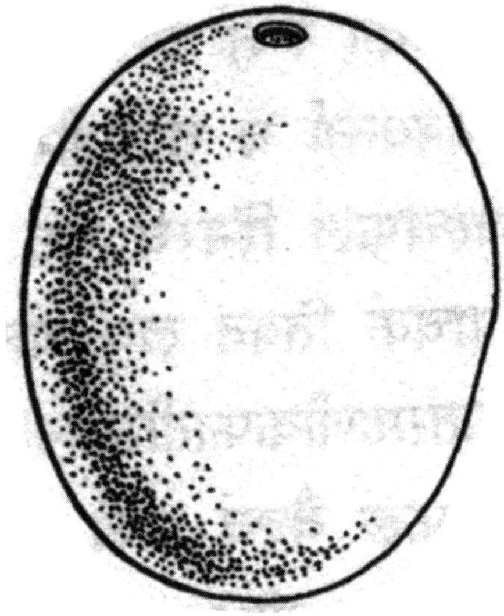

Fig 6.2 Fruit of bael

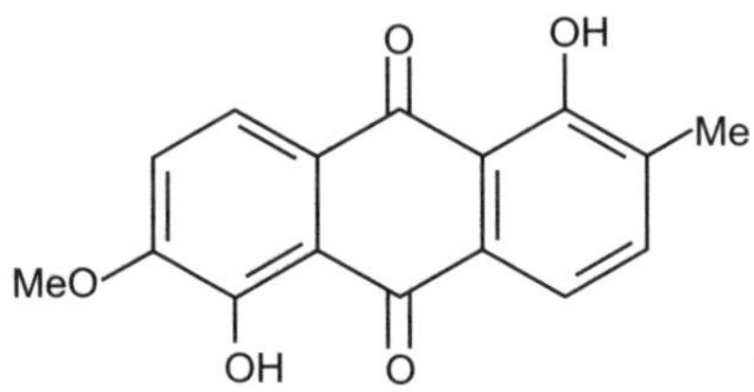

Marmesin

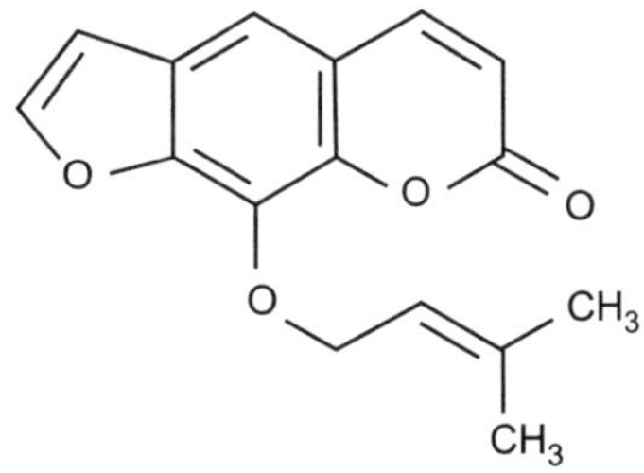

Imperatorin

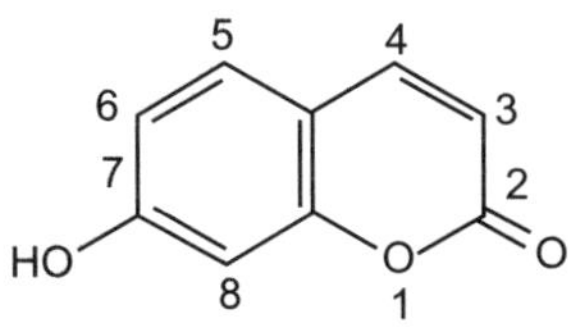

Umbelliferone

Uses

- The raw fruits are used to treat chronic diarrhoea and dysentery, while ripe ones are used as laxative.
- The fruits relieve flatulence, acidity and irritable bowel syndrome.
- The roots are dipped in neem oil and used to treat ear problems.
- The infusion is used to treat peptic ulcer.

Note: If taken continually, the fruit can cause loss of normal elasticity of the intestines, leading to flatulence.

6.4 RASNA

Common name : Lesser galangal

Biological source : Rhizome of *Alpinia officinarum* obtained from plants that are 4–10 years of age; washed, trimmed and cut into segments and carefully dried. It consists of not less than 0.5% of volatile oils.

Family : Zingiberaceae

Morphology

Form : Cylindrical, irregularly branched and bent

Size : 5–10 cm long and up to 2 cm thick

Colour : Copper red on the outside and cinnamon brown inside

Surface : Marked with fine, light coloured annuli

Odour : Aromatic

Taste : Characteristic, spicy, aromatic and pungent

Fracture : Fibrous and tough

Chemical constituents: Essential oils (0.5%–1%), cineole, α-pinene, eugenol, sesquiterpenes and sesquiterpene alocohols; alpinol resins or gelangol; tannins, phlobaphenes and flavanoids—kaempferol and galangin, a dioxyflavonol. The active principles are the volatile oils and resins.

Uses

- It is a carminative, stomachic and stimulant; therefore, used in treating flatulence, dyspepsia, vomiting and sea sickness.
- It is useful in relieving fever.
- It is an anti-rheumatic.
- It also has anti-bacterial and anti-fungal properties.

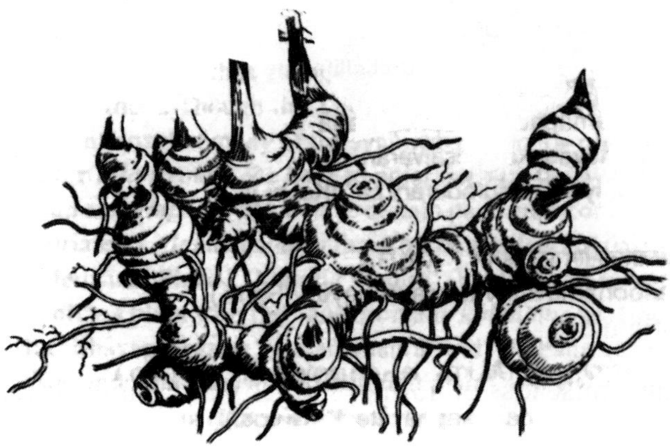

Fig 6.3 Rhizomes of rasna

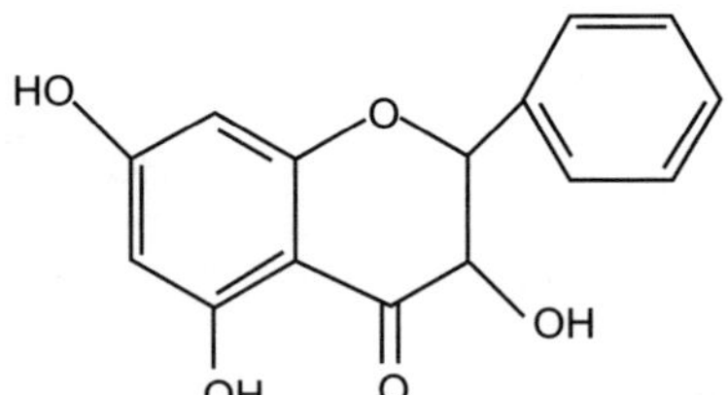

Galangin

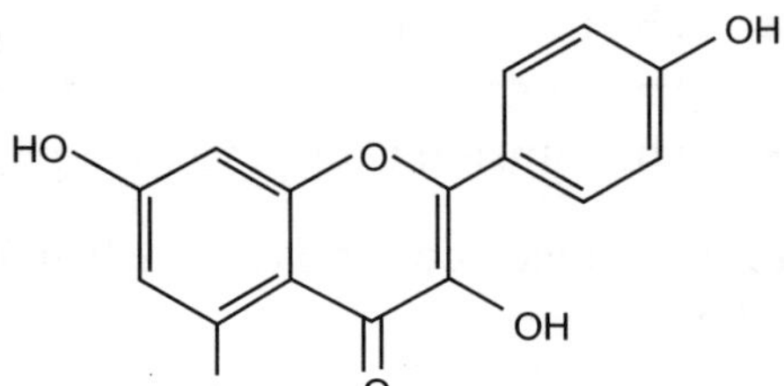

Kaempferol

6.5 GUDUCHI

Common name : Gulbel, Madhuparni, Amritha
Biological source : Stems and roots of *Tinospora cordifolia*
Family : Menispermaceae
Morphology

Plant : Climber shrub
Leaves : Heart-shaped at base, broadly ovate or orbicular
Stem : Light grey, paper-like, about 6 cm in diameter
Flowers : Small, greenish-yellow, found as racemes 7–14 cm long
Fruits : Red

Chemical constituents: Diterpenoids such as thiosporide, tinosporide and columbin; sesquiterpenes like tinocordifolioside; alkaloids, berberine and jatrorhizine

Uses

- When applied externally, it is highly effective in treating gout and skin diseases.
- It is rejuvenative, bestows longevity, improves health and imparts good complexion.
- It is used for treating digestive problems such as hyperacidity, colitis, abdominal pain, vomiting and loss of appetite.
- It is used in the treatment of hepatitis.
- The bitter tonic is used to treat problems arising from disturbed pitta.
- The starch (sattva) of guduchi is traditionally used to treat chronic fever. It is also used as an appetizer.

Note: For best results guduchi should be used fresh.

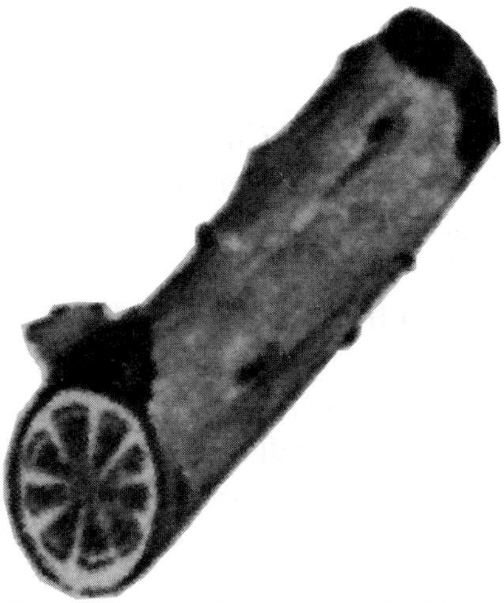

Fig 6.4 Stem and root of guduchi

6.6 KALIJEERA

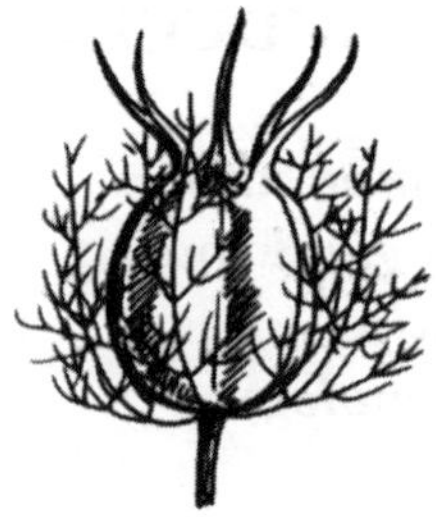

Fig. 6.5 Seeds of kalijeera

Common name : Black cumin, *Kalonji*
Biological source : Ripe seeds of *Nigella sativa*
Family : Ranunculaceae
Morphology

Plant : Herb, 20–30 cm long
Leaves : Pinnate and linearly lanceolate
Flowers : Light blue and white with 5–10 petals, on solitary, long peduncles
Fruits : Huge, inflated capsule made up of 3–7 united follicles, each having large number of seeds
Seeds : Black, trigonous, contain volatile oil with unpleasant odour

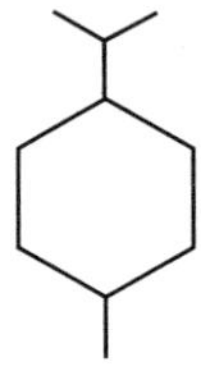

Nigellone

Chemical constituents: Volatile oils with an unpleasant odour, carvone, d-limonene, cyamine and nigellone

Uses

- It is widely used for respiratory ailments such as asthma and bronchitis.
- It promotes digestion.
- It improves working of the kidneys and liver.
- It is used in disorders of the circulatory system.
- It has anti-rheumatic and anti-inflammatory properties.
- It is a galactogogue.
- It is used as an anti-parasitic.
- The oil is used in the treatment of boils and eczema.

6.7 GOKHRU

Common name : *Gokshura*, Land Caltrops, Puncture vine
Biological source : Fruits of *Tribulus terrestris*
Family : Zygophyllaceae
Morphology

Plant : Annual herb with prostrate or diffused stems; flexible branches with silky hairs
Leaves : Pari-pinnate, with 6–7 pairs of leaflets arranged elliptically
Flowers : Yellow, solitary and axillary
Fruits : Globose, with five hairy cocci, each with two very long sharp rigid spines, many shorter spines; surface of the fruit is covered with many hairs.
Seeds : Numerous in each coccus, separated by transverse partitions

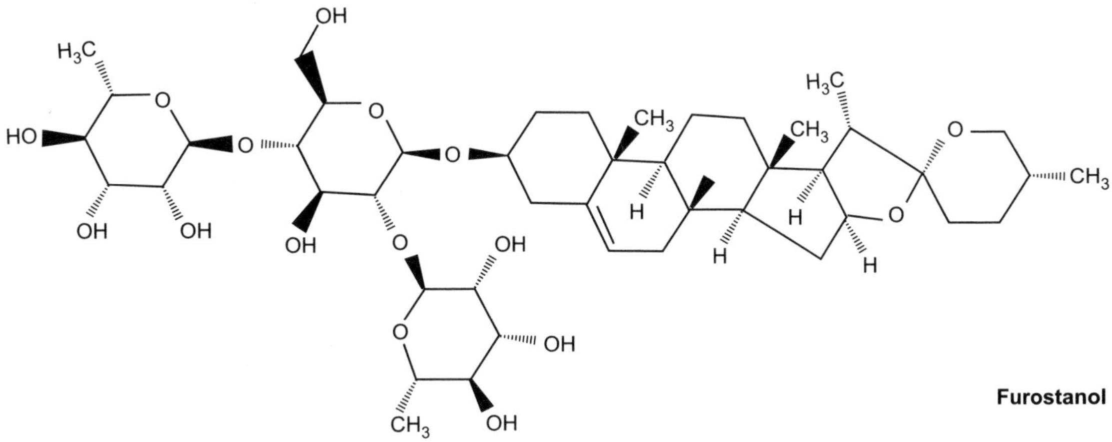

Furostanol

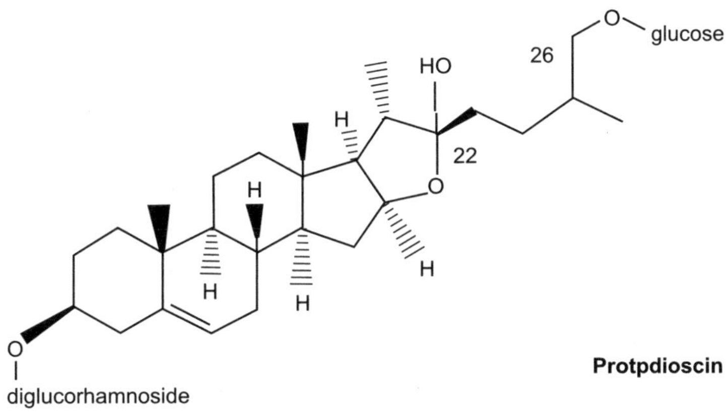

Protpdioscin

Chemical constituents: Steroid saponins and steroid sapogenins, furostanol glycosides —protodioscin which gives spirostanol and diosgenin on acid hydrolysis; small quantities of lipogenin, glucose and rhamnose, hecogenin and neotigogenin

Uses

- It is a coolant and an emollient.
- It is used as an appetite stimulant in anorexia.
- It is effective in dyspepsia.
- It has laxative properties.
- It is a cardiotonic and styptic.
- Due to its lithotriptic properties, it is used in treating gall bladder and kidney stones.
- It is useful in cough and asthma.
- The plant ash is used externally for relieving arthritic pain.

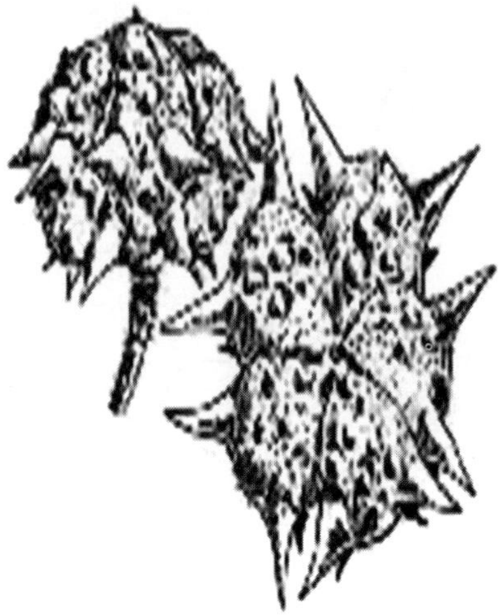

Fig 6.6 Fruits of gokhru

6.8 SHILAJIT

Biological source

It is a herbo-mineral drug ejected out of fissures in the iron-rich rocks during summer. In the raw form, it is a bituminous substance, which is a compact mass of vegetable organic matter composed of dark red gummy matrix. It is bitter in taste, and smells like stale urine of the cow. The botanical name of shilajit is *Asphaltum* (mineral pitch).

It occurs naturally in the Himalayas, Vindhyas and other mountains of India and Nepal. Before purification, shilajit is a hard, brownish black to dark, greasy, black resin with a distinctive smell and taste.

Colour

Iron shilajit : Blackish brown
Copper shilajit : Blue
Silver shilajit : White
Gold Shilajit : Red

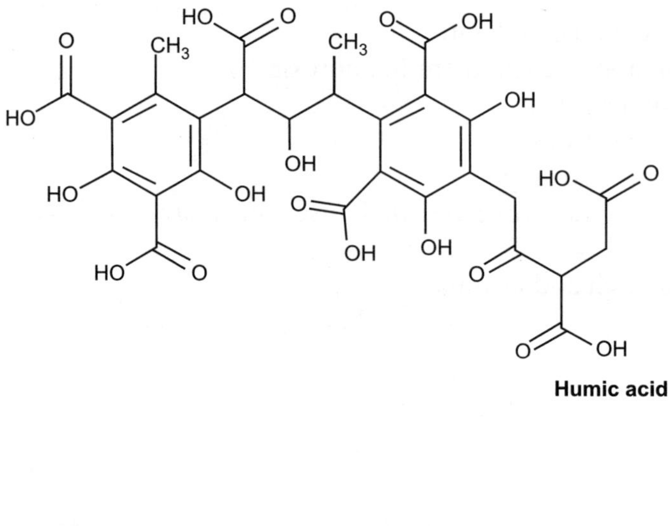

Humic acid

Chemical constituents: Aluminoids, fatty acid, trace elements, waxes, minerals, methoxy carboxy biphenyls; humic acid and fulvic acid

Uses

- It is anti-diabetic and hence improves pancreatic functioning and regulates blood sugar levels.
- It helps in reducing fat and aids weight loss.
- It promotes uptake of minerals like phosphorus, calcium and magnesium into tissues and muscles.
- It is a blood purifier.
- It has immune stimulant effect.
- It is considered an aphrodisiac.

6.9 ARJUNA

Common name : *Koha*, white marudah
Biological source : Dried bark of *Terminalia arjuna*
Family : Combretaceae
Morphology

Plant : Large, evergreen, deciduous tree about 85 feet long
Bark : Grey and smooth outer surface; striated and red inner surface
Leaves : Conical, pale brown on lower surface and dull green on the upper
Flowers : Yellow
Shape : Flat, slightly curved
Size : About 15 cm long, 10 cm wide and 1 cm thick
Colour : Ash coloured on the outer side but reddish and striated on the inner side
Fracture : Fibrous

Chemical constituents: Tannins (12%), pyrocatechol tannins, large amount of calcium salts and traces of aluminium and magnesium salts; arjuna glycosides, phytosterols, organic acids and organic esters, saponin-like substance, sugars and colouring matter.

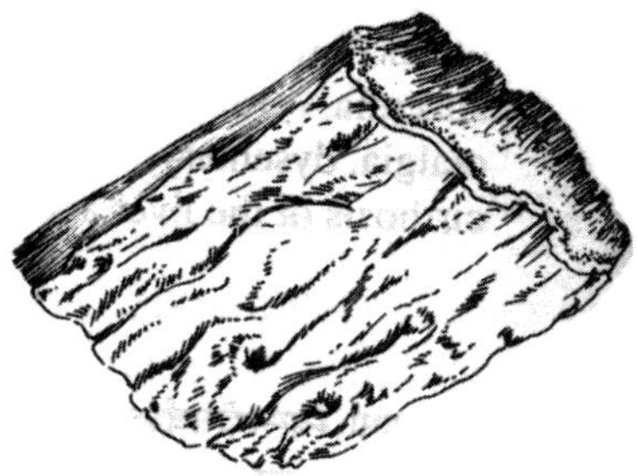

Fig 6.7 Dried bark of arjuna

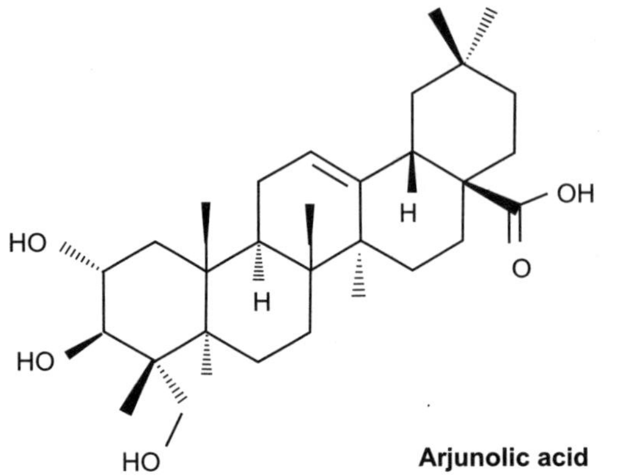

Arjunolic acid

Uses

- It has traditionally been used in cardiac problems (angina pectoris), hypertension and hypercholesterolemia; its effects are probably due to the anti-oxidant action of the chemical constituents.
- It is protective in gastric ulcers.
- It is effective in the treatment of sexually transmitted diseases like gonorrhea.

6.10 CHIRATA

Common name : Indian Gentian, *Bhunimba*

Biological source : Whole plant of *Swertia chirata* collected in flowering stage and dried

Family : Gentianaceae

Morphology

Stem : Glabrous, with continuous pith, dark purplish brown

Leaves : Opposite, ovate, lanceolate, glabrous, entire

Roots : Short, oblique and stout

Fruits : Bicarpellary but unilocular, with numerous tiny brownish seeds

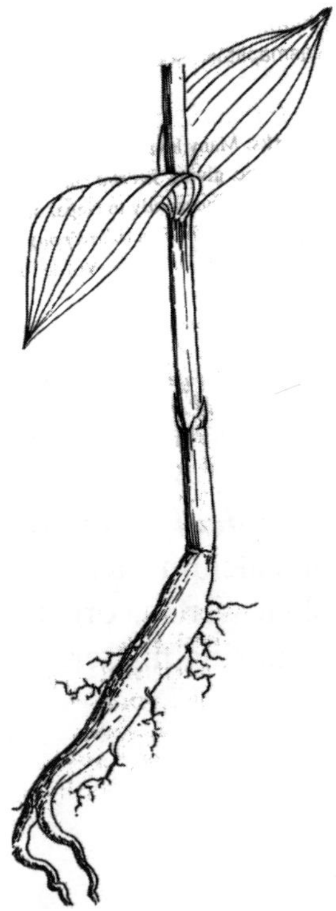

Fig 6.8 Stem of chirata

Chemical constituents: The main constituents are the two bitter principles, ophelic acid and chiratin. The latter occurs in greater quantity and on acid hydrolysis, yields chiratogenin and ophelic acid. Neither ophelic acid nor chiratin has been obtained in crystals. Amarogentin, a glycoside, is also present.

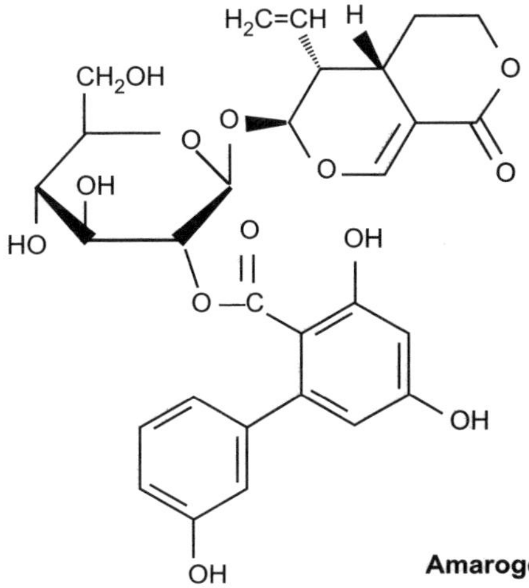

Amarogentin

Uses

- It is used as an appetizer in dyspepsia.
- It is also used as a febrifuge.

6.11 TYLOPHORA

Common name : Indian Ipecac, Antamul
Biological source : Fresh and dried material of *Tylophora indica*
Family : Asclepiadaceae
Morphology

Plant : Small and slender perennial climber.
Leaves : Ovate-oblong to elliptic-oblong, acute to acuminate, cordate at base, thick, pubescent beneath when young, glabrous above
Flowers : Tiny, 1–1.5 cm across, in 2- to 3-flowered fascicles in axillary umbellate cymes
Roots : Fleshy and long, bark is pale brown with longitudinal fissures
Fracture : Brittle

Chemical constituents: Alkaloids like tylophorine, tylophorinine, tylophorinidine, septicine and isotylocrebrine; tannins, saponins and flavonoids

Uses

- The leaves and roots have emetic, laxative and expectorant action.
- It is used for treating allergies, hay fever, cold, bronchial asthma and dermatitis.
- It is a blood purifier.
- The powder of the root or leaf is used to treat diarrhoea, dysentery and intermittent fever.

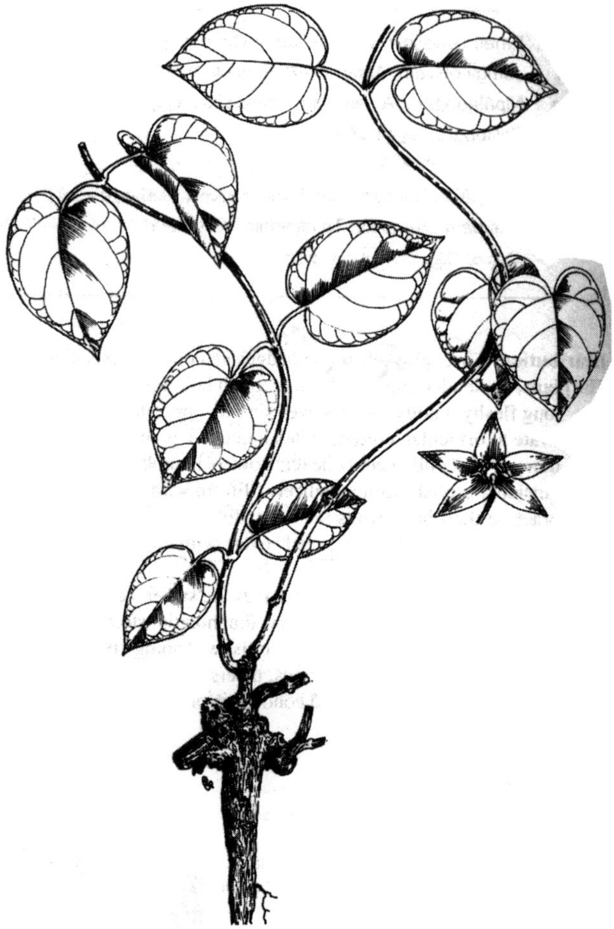

Fig. 6.9 Whole plant of tylophora

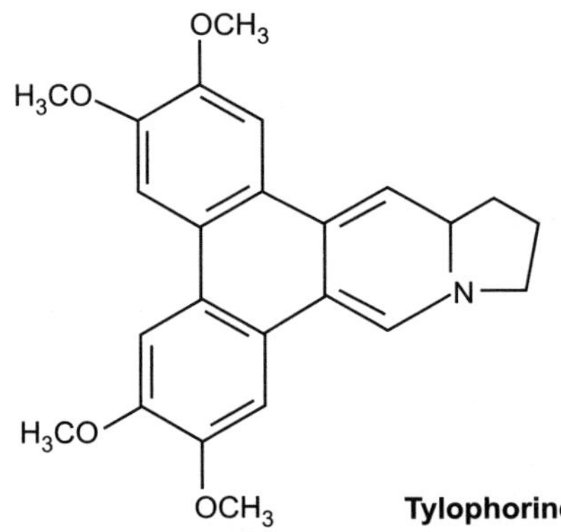

Tylophorine

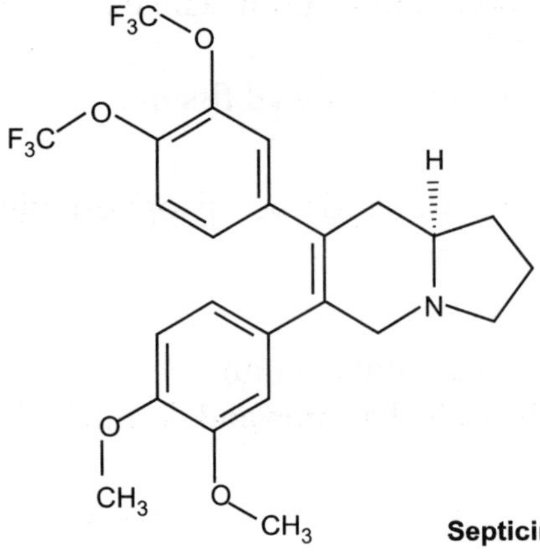

Septicine

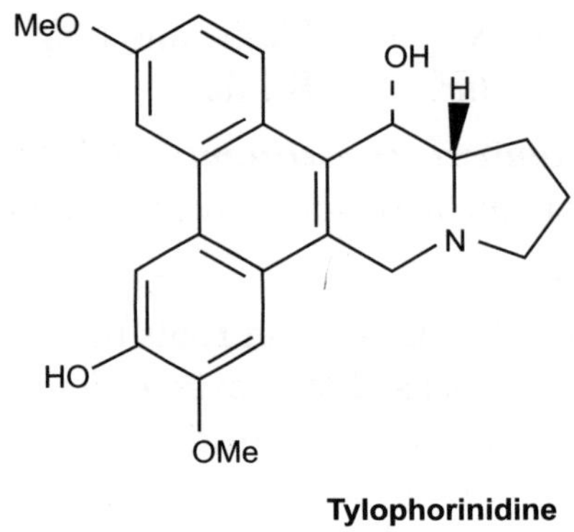

Tylophorinidine

6.12 APAMARGA

Common name : Prickly chaff flower, Chirchidi
Biological source : Dried whole plant of *Achyranthes aspera*
Family : Amaranthaceae
Morphology

Plant : Annual or perennial herb, with a woody base, 30–90 cm tall

Stem : Yellowish brown, erect and branched, cylindrical, hairy, solid up to 60 cm long.

Leaves : Petiolate, alternate, elliptical or suborbicular, acute entire pubescent above and usually white and hairy underneath

Flowers : Greenish white, numerous in axillary or terminal spikes; bract and bracteole persisting and ending in spine

Roots : Long, cylindrical main root with thick secondary and tertiary roots

Chemical constituents: Ecdysone, ecdysterone, inokosterone, triterpenoid saponins containing oleonelic acid as an aglycone. Alkaloids like achyranthine and betaine are present along with water-soluble bases and saponin glycosides C and D.

Uses

- It is effective in treating abdominal and liver disorders.
- It is a blood purifier.
- It has astringent and diuretic properties.
- Plant decoction is used in pneumonia and dropsy.
- It is an anti-cancer agent.

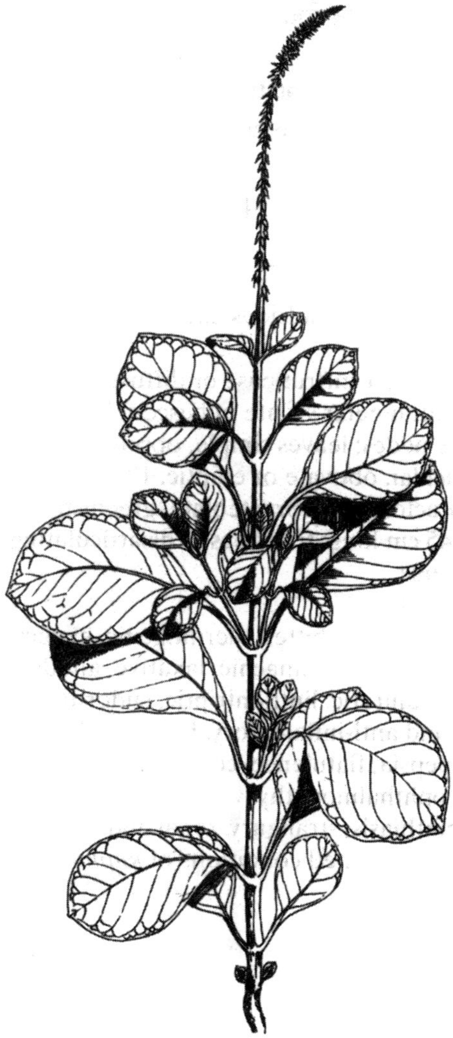

Fig. 6.10 Whole plant of apamarga

6.13 SHANKHPUSHPI

Common name : Dwarf morning glory, Shankhahuli
Biological source : Aerial parts of *Evolvulus alsinoides* and *Convolvulus pluricaulis*
Family : Convulvulaceae
Morphology

Plant : Small, diffuse perennial herb, highly branched and hairy
Leaves : Sessile, 2.5–4 cm long, lanceolate and decussate with 3 prominent vertical lines, densely covered with silky hair
Flowers : Axillary white (*C. pluricaulis*) or light blue (*E. alsinoides*) and mostly solitary in the upper axils
Roots : Greenish-white, branched with secondary roots 1–5 cm long and 0.1–0.4 cm thick.
Fruits : Globose, 4-valve capsules and small

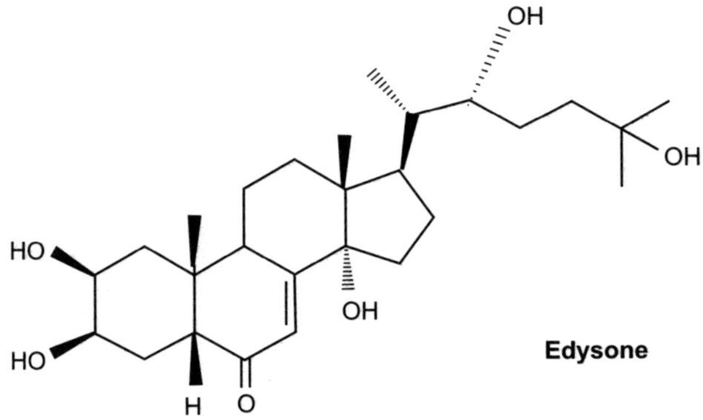

Edysone

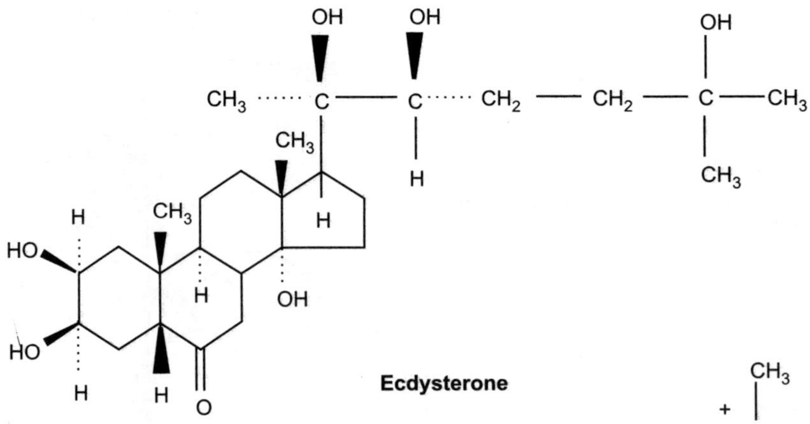

Ecdysterone

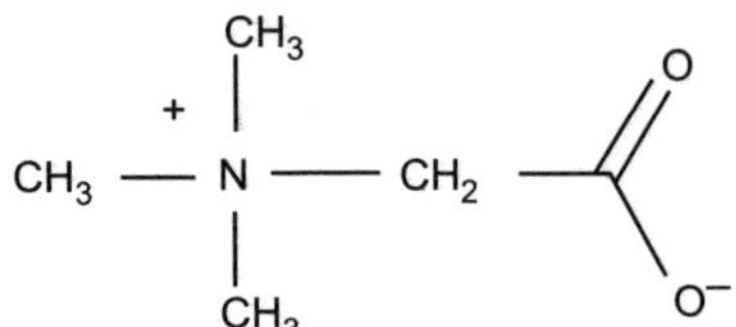

Betaine

Chemical constituents: The plant contains an alkaloid called shankhapushpine. The fresh plant contains volatile oil and potassium chloride. It also contains a neutral fat, an organic acid and saline substances. Alkaloids like evolvine and betaine have been isolated.

Uses

All parts of the plant are used for medicinal purposes.

- The medicated oil is used externally as a hair tonic; it is also said to prevent hair loss and premature greying.
- A paste of the plant is used topically for various skin diseases.
- It is widely used as a brain tonic and for treating various neurological conditions such as memory loss, nervous debility and dementia.
- The fresh juice of the plant is used as an appetite stimulant, mild laxative and anti-flatulent.
- It is used as a diuretic in hypertension and urinary disorders.
- It is an aphrodisiac and promotes fertility in women.
- It is a general tonic and rejuvenative.
- It is an anti-viral agent against Ranikhet disease virus.

Exercises

Short answers

1. Discuss the biological source, family, chemical constituents and uses of guduchi, arjuna and shatavari.
2. List the chemical constituents present in rasna, shankhapushpi and gokhru.
3. Write a note on chirata and apamarga.
4. Give the biological source and uses of any one drug belonging to the following families: Amaranthaceae, Rutaceae, Menispermaceae and Asclepiadaceae
5. Give the uses of chirata, tylophora, apamarga and shilajit.

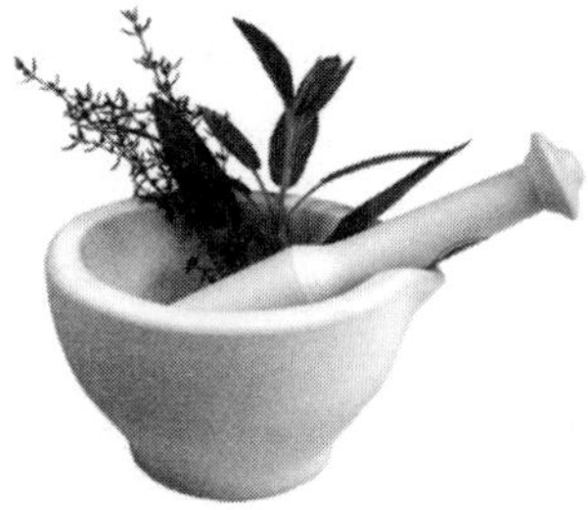

7

Isolation of Compounds from Natural Sources

In This Chapter, You Will Learn

- The common methods of isolation of important natural drugs
- The factors to be considered in choosing the method of isolation
- The methods of quantitative estimation and identification tests for a few important drugs.

Plants contain various chemical compounds. While some of them occur in all cells and are necessary for metabolism and reproduction, others form cellular components. A few compounds known as secondary metabolites are characteristic of a particular species and possess distinct pharmacological properties. These compounds can be isolated and utilized in the prevention or cure of diseases or disorders. A wide range of methods such as digestion, maceration, percolation and solvent extraction are useful in the process of extracting active ingredients from plant sources.

Choosing the right method of isolation

The most important factor for deciding the method of isolation is the nature of the compound to be isolated. The general features that are considered include solubility (hydrophilicity and hydrophobicity), charge, acid–base properties, stability and molecular size. Depending on the chemical properties of the functional groups and moieties contained in the compounds, such as, aldehydes, phenols, alcohols, acids and alkalies, chemical derivatization techniques may be adopted to convert the component into a derivative form. Such derivatives are of a different physical and chemical nature and can hence be subsequently isolated from the mixture and then reconverted back to the original form by another reaction.

7.1 QUININE

Quinine is an important alkaloid of cinchona bark. It belongs to the quinoline group of alkaloids. It is a stereoisomer of quinidine, and has anti-malarial, anti-pyretic, analgesic and anti-inflammatory properties.

Biological source

It is obtained from the dried bark of *Cinchona officinalis*, *Cinchona succirubra*, *Cinchona ledgeriana* and *Cinchona calisaya* belonging to the Rubiaceae family.

Isolation

The bark material is taken as a dry powder and mixed well with about 30% of its weight of calcium hydroxide [$Ca(OH)_2$] or calcium oxide (CaO) and sufficient quantity of 5% sodium hydroxide (NaOH) solution to make a paste. This is allowed to stand for a few hours to liberate the free alkaloids. The mass is then transferred to a Soxhlet apparatus and the alkaloids are extracted with benzene. Subsequently, the benzene extract is shaken with successive portions of 5% sulphuric acid (H_2SO_4) to convert the alkaloid bases into water-soluble alkaloidal sulphate salts. The pH of the aqueous acid extract is adjusted to 6.5 with dilute NaOH. The extract is cooled and allowed to stand. Crystals of neutral quinine sulphate are separated from cinchonine and cinchonidine by repeated crystallization from hot water. The colouring matter is removed by the use of activated charcoal.

The crystals of quinine sulphate are dissolved in dilute H_2SO_4 and the solution is made alkaline with ammonia. Initially, amorphous quinine is formed, which later changes into a crystalline form. It is finally washed to remove sodium and ammonium salts and dried at 45–55°C.

Tests for identification

- A dilute solution of quinine or a quinine salt in dilute H_2SO_4 gives a characteristic blue fluorescence.

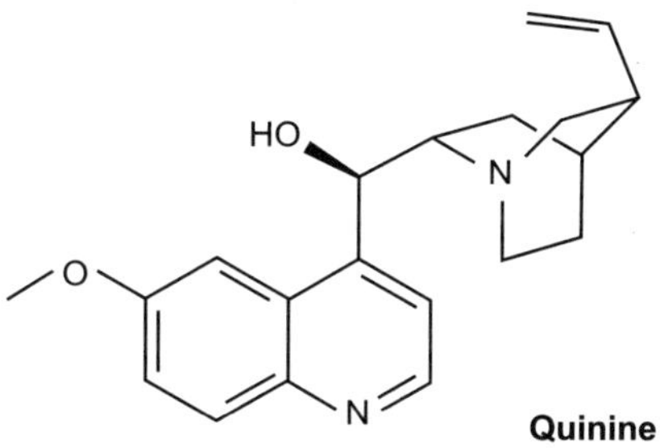

Quinine

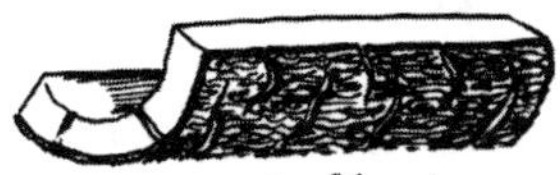

Fig. 7.1 Bark of cinchona

- ***Thalleioquin test*** To 2–3 ml of a weakly acidic solution of a quinine salt, a few drops of bromine water and then 0.5–1 ml of strong ammonia are added. A characteristic emerald green colour is produced, due to the formation of a product called thalleioquin; its constitution is not known. Quinidine answers this test, while cinchonine and cinchonidine do not respond.
- Quinine gives a white precipitate with silver nitrate ($AgNO_3$) solution.
- Identification by thin layer chromatography (TLC)

Adsorbent	:	Silica gel
Solvent system	:	Chloroform and diethyl amine (9:1)
Detection	:	Spraying with methanolic sulphuric acid (10%) or by UV light

Estimation

Fluorimetry

Quinine can be assayed by the measurement of the blue fluorescence (366 nm) produced by irradiation in dilute H_2SO_4 solution at 450 nm. For estimation, a stock solution is prepared by dissolving 10 mg of quinine sulphate in 100 ml of dilute H_2SO_4. Serial dilutions are subsequently prepared by using 0.1N H_2SO_4. The fluorescence is measured and a standard graph of fluorescence versus concentration is plotted. The amount of quinine in the unknown sample is estimated by measuring its fluorescence and interpolating from the standard graph.

Non-aqueous titration

0.2 g of quinine sulphate is dissolved in 20 ml of chloroform and 20 ml of acetic anhydride. This is then estimated by potentiometric titration with 0.1M perchloric acid. A blank should be performed to make necessary corrections.

7.2 EPHEDRINE

Ephedrine is a sympathomimetic alkaloid obtained from various plants of the genus Ephedra. It has decongestant and appetite suppressant properties and is also used to treat hypotension arising from the administration of anesthesia.

Biological source

The dried aerial parts of *Ephedra sinica* and *Ephedra equisetina* belonging to family Ephedraceae (Gnetaceae) are the main source.

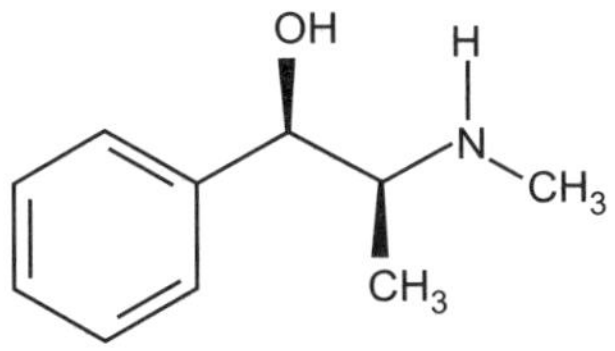

Ephedrine

ISOLATION

It was first isolated by Nagai in 1887. In this procedure, Ephedra powder is made alkaline with sodium carbonate (Na_2CO_3) and then macerated with benzene overnight. The benzene layer is separated by filtration and then treated with dilute HCl to convert the alkaloids into salts. The aqueous layer is separated and made alkaline with solid potassium carbonate (K_2CO_3). This treatment liberates free alkaloid bases. Subsequently, these alkaloidal bases are extracted with chloroform. The chloroform extract is evaporated to get the residue. This is mixed with oxalic acid solution and warmed. The alkaloidal oxalates formed include ephedrine oxalate and pseudo-ephedrine oxalate. The former, being less soluble in cold water, crystallizes on cooling, whereas the latter remains in solution.

Ephedrine is liberated from its oxalate by shaking with alkali solution and then extracted with a mixture of chloroform and ether (1:3) to get ephedrine.

TESTS FOR IDENTIFICATION

- Ephedrine is dissolved in water and dilute HCl is then added and tested separately with 10% copper sulphate ($CuSO_4$)solution and 20% NaOH solution. A purple or violet colour develops. This is extractable with ether. On shaking with ether, the organic layer becomes purple, whereas the aqueous layer turns blue.
- A slightly alkaline solution of ephedrine on warming with ninhydrin turns violet.
- Ephedrine gives pink to red colouration with concentrated H_2SO_4 and 3–4 drops of 40% formaldehyde (HCHO).

ESTIMATION

IP 96 method

0.5 g of the sample is accurately weighed and dissolved in 5 ml of 95% ethanol. 50 ml of 0.1M HCl is added and titrated with 0.1M NaOH, using methyl red as the indicator, until a yellow colour is produced.

Non-aqueous titration method

0.17 g of an accurately weighed sample is dissolved in 10 ml of mercuric acetate solution, by warming gently. 50 ml of acetone is added and titrated with 0.1M perchloric acid. The end point is determined potentiometrically.

Fluorimetry
The sample is treated with dansyl chloride and the absorbance is measured at 366 nm.

7.3 DIOSGENIN

Diosgenin is a steroidal compound obtained by hydrolysis of saponins by acids, strong bases or enzymes. The saponins are extracted from Dioscorea tubers. The aglycone diosgenin is used for the commercial synthesis of cortisone, pregnenolone, progesterone and other steroidal compounds.

BIOLOGICAL SOURCE

The main sources are the rhizomes of various species of Dioscorea like *Dioscorea deltoidea*, *Dioscorea composita* and *Dioscorea floribunda* belonging to the family Dioscoreaceae. Other sources include the rhizome of *Costus speciosus* (Zingiberaceae) and the seeds of *Trigonella foenum graecum* (Leguminosae)

ISOLATION

Diosgenin can be isolated from the rhizome by extraction with a solvent followed by hydrolysis to remove sugar moieties. This liberates the sapogenin which is then made alkaline, isolated and purified to obtain pure diosgenin. The various methods available are discussed below.

Alcohol extraction method
The finely powdered drug is extracted with either methanol or ethanol and the extract is concentrated. This extract is then hydrolyzed with 2N HCl for 2–12 hours. The residue containing diosgenin is collected by filtration and further purified by recrystallization from an organic solvent such as benzene, hexane or alcohol.

This method has the following disadvantages:

- Unsaturated sapogenin quickly decomposes to spirostadiene.
- A gummy material is formed alongside.
- It is time consuming.

These shortcomings can be overcome by treating the hydrolyzed extract with lime or other alkalis to remove phenolic and coloured impurities.

Acid hydrolysis method
The powdered drug is refluxed with 2N or 4N mineral acid in an autoclave for 2–6 hours. It is filtered and the hydrolysate is washed with lime and then with water to make it neutral. This is then dried and the dried product is extracted exhaustively with a hydrocarbon solvent like petroleum ether or toluene for 6 hours. The extract is concentrated to get crystals of diosgenin.

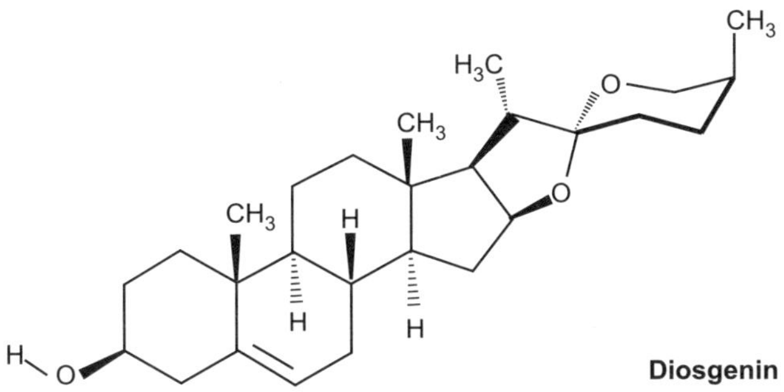

Diosgenin

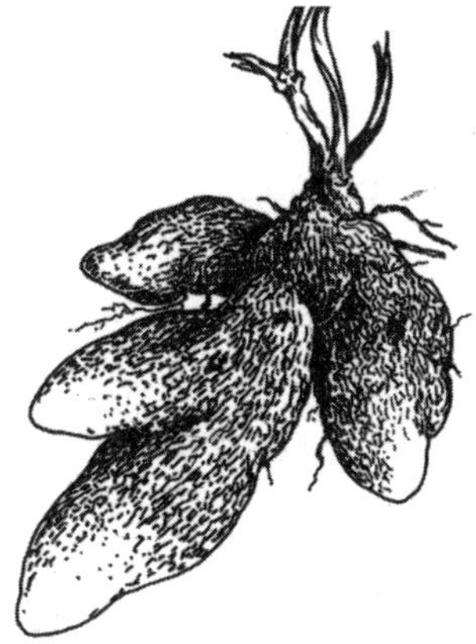

Fig. 7.2 Rhizomes of Dioscorea

This method has the following advantages:

- It is less time consuming.
- A purer compound can be obtained.
- It is easy to perform.
- No gummy material is formed.

Fermentation-cum-acid hydrolysis method

The powdered drug is subjected to fermentation for two days, it is then dried by spreading in the sun until the moisture content is reduced to 7%–8%. The dried drug is then hydrolyzed with a mineral acid, neutralized with lime and water and the acid-free hydrolyzed mass is extracted with heptane.

Estimation

The methods of estimation include gravimetry, spectrophotometry, gas–liquid chromatography (GLC), IR spectroscopy, high performance liquid chromatography (HPLC) and HPTLC.

High pressure thin layer chromatography (HPTLC) method

The standard solution is prepared in chloroform. One gram of the drug is refluxed with 25 ml of 2.5N HCl for about four hours, and cooled and filtered through Whatman filter paper. The residue is washed with water until free from acid, and then dried at less than 80°C in an oven. This is then extracted with petroleum ether using a Soxhlet apparatus for about four hours, evaporated to dryness and the residue is dissolved in 5 ml of chloroform. The volume is then made up to 10 ml with chloroform and further dilutions can be made if necessary.

The solvent system used is toluene and ethyl acetate (7:3).

Procedure Known volumes of standard and sample are applied in triplicate on precoated HPTLC plates. The plates are developed to a distance of 8 cm. The plate is air dried and sprayed with Lieberman–Burchard reagent and heated at 120°C until the spot corresponding to diosgenin turns black (about 15 minutes).

TLC method

Adsorbent	:	Silica gel 60
Solvent system	:	Toluene and ethyl acetate (7:3)
Reference standard	:	1 mg of diosgenin in 1 ml of chloroform

Sample preparation The powdered drug is refluxed with 50 ml of 10% HCl for two hours. The residue is washed with 20 ml of dilute Na_2CO_3 solution and then with water. The residue is later extracted with three portions of 25 ml of solvent ether and the ether extracts are combined. This is concentrated to obtain a residue which is then dissolved in 2 ml of chloroform.

Procedure 20 µml of test and reference solutions are applied in two different tracks on a pre-coated silica gel 60 plate of uniform thickness (0.2 mm). The spots are visualized by spraying with anisaldehyde sulphuric acid reagent.

Evaluation In daylight, a dark green spot develops with R_f value of 0.37, corresponding to diosgenin in both reference and test solution tracks. The sample also shows a violet spot (R_f: 0.96, 0.45) and a green spot (R_f: 0.91, 0.27, 0.09).

Gas liquid chromatography method

Column	:	Chromosorb 80–100 mesh
Carrier gas	:	Nitrogen 5 ml/min
Temperature	:	270°C, outlet 230°C

Column maintained at 250°C

Detector	:	Photodiode detector
Retention time	:	20 minutes

7.4 SENNOSIDES

The sennosides A, B, C and D are dimeric glycosides of senna. These are hydroxy-anthracene glycosides obtained from the leaves in the form of calcium salts.

Biological source

Senna consists of dried leaflets of *Cassia angustifolia* and *Cassia acutifolia* belonging to the Leguminosae family.

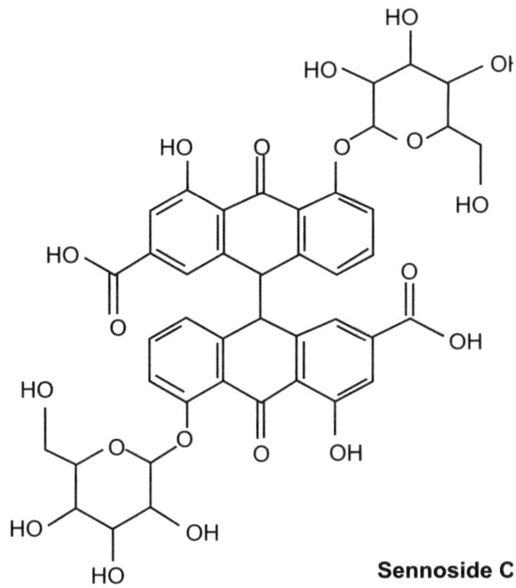

Sennoside C

Isolation

Sennosides can be isolated by various methods—Ahmed and Samia method, Stoll and Becker method, modified Stoll and Becker method, Notherman and Lic method, Mauzaram et al method and extracted as calcium salts. The last method, the calcium sennoside method is preferred since the products have better stability than those obtained from the other methods.

The powdered leaves are extracted with benzene for two hours on an electric shaker and then filtered; the marc is collected and dried. The dried marc is then extracted with 70% methanol for four hours and the methanol extract is collected. The marc is again extracted with methanol. The above two extracts are combined and the volume is reduced to 1/8 of the original volume. This concentrated extract is then acidified to a pH of 3.2 with dilute HCl and set aside at a temperature of 50°C for two hours. It is then filtered and anhydrous calcium chloride in rectified spirit is added to the filtrate. The pH is adjusted to 8 by adding ammonia and it is set aside for two hours. The precipitate of calcium sennosides is collected and dried.

Tests for identification

Borntrager's Test

The powdered leaves are boiled with dilute H_2SO_4 and the filtrate is collected and cooled. It is shaken with an organic solvent like benzene, chloroform and carbon tetrachloride. The organic layer is separated and an equal quantity of ammonia is added. The ammonia layer turns pink to red, indicating the presence of anthraquinone glycosides (sennosides) in the drug.

TLC

For identifying sennosides by TLC, the following parameters are adopted.

Adsorbent	:	Silica gel 60 P 254
Solvent system	:	*n*-propanol, ethyl acetate and water (4:4:3)
Detection	:	Nitric acid/potassium hydroxide reagent or visible/UV 366 nm
Sample preparation	:	One gram of the powdered drug is extracted with 5 ml methanol by heating on a water bath, for 15 minutes. This is then filtered and the filtrate is used for spotting.
Visualization		
Daylight	:	7–9 red-brown zones
UV 366 nm	:	Same zones–lemon yellow or light blue

R_f value for the system

Sennoside A: 0.4

Sennoside B: 0.2

Sennoside C: 0.7

Sennoside D: 0.5

Estimation

IP 96 method

The estimation is done by colorimetry. The procedure involves extraction, removal of the free anthraquinone genins, oxidative cleavage of dianthrones, acid hydrolysis to give monomeric anthraquinone genins and finally, colorimetric determination based on Borntrager's test.

Procedure About 0.15 g of fine senna powder is mixed with 30 ml of water and the weight is noted. It is refluxed on a water bath for 15 minutes, cooled and weighed. Water is added to restore the weight to the previous level. The solution is centrifuged and 20 ml of the supernatant liquid is taken into a separating funnel. Then, 0.1 ml of 2M HCl is added and the sennosides are extracted by shaking well with three successive 15 ml portions of chloroform. The chloroform layer is discarded and the aqueous layer is mixed with 0.1 g of sodium bicarbonate. After shaking for 3 minutes and centrifuging, 10 ml of the supernatant liquid is taken in a round-bottomed flask with a ground glass stopper. 20 ml of ferric chloride solution is added and refluxed on a water bath for 20 minutes with shaking until the precipitate is dissolved. This solution is cooled and transferred to a separating funnel. It is shaken with three 25 ml portions of ether. The ether extracts are combined, washed with water and diluted to 100 ml with ether. 10 ml of the extract is evaporated to dryness. The dry residue is dissolved in 10 ml of 0.5% magnesium acetate in methanol. Absorbance of the pink colour obtained at 515 nm is measured using methanol as a blank. The percentage content of hydroxy anthracene glycosides is calculated and expressed as Sennoside B, taking 240 as the value of A (1%, 1 cm) at 515 nm.

7.5 GLYCYRRHIZIN

It is the active constituent of glycyrrhiza (liquorice). It is responsible for the sweet taste of the drug. Glycyrrhizin is the potassium or calcium salt of glycyrrhizinic (or glycyrrhizic) acid. Glycyrrhizinic acid is a glycoside, which on hydrolysis gives 18 β-glycyyrhetic acid (glycyrrhetinic acid). Glycyrrhetic acid has a triterpenoid structure.

Biological source

The peeled or unpeeled roots and stolons of *Glycyrrhiza glabra* belonging to the Leguminosae family are the main source of glycyrrhiza.

Isolation

The methods for isolation are based on the solubility of glycyrrhizin. It is readily soluble in hot water and alcohol, but slightly soluble in cold water; it is insoluble in ether. The three methods of isolation are:

- Acid precipitation method
- Alcohol extraction method
- Ammonium extraction method

Acid precipitation method

In this method glycyrrhizin is precipitated from an aqueous solution by the addition of concentrated H_2SO_4 or HCl to adjust the pH to 2.8. 50 g of glycyrrhiza is weighed and boiled with 300 ml of water in a beaker. The supernatant liquid is decanted, the remaining residue is filtered and the filtrate is collected. The decanted supernatant liquid is also filtered, the filtrate is collected and both the filtrates are combined. The pH is adjusted to 2.8 by the addition of acid, and the glycyrrhizin precipitates out. This is filtered and the precipitate is collected, washed with cold water to free it from acid and transferred to a china dish. It is then heated gently to remove the water content and obtain a shiny brown mass of glycyrrhizin.

Alcohol extraction method

The insolubility of glycyrrhizin in non-polar solvents can be utilized for removing interfering substances. Alcohol is used for extraction. After removing the interfering substances, the alcoholic extract is successively extracted with various solvents of increasing polarity to remove the interfering substances. Finally, by concentrating the alcoholic extract, glycyrrhizin is isolated.

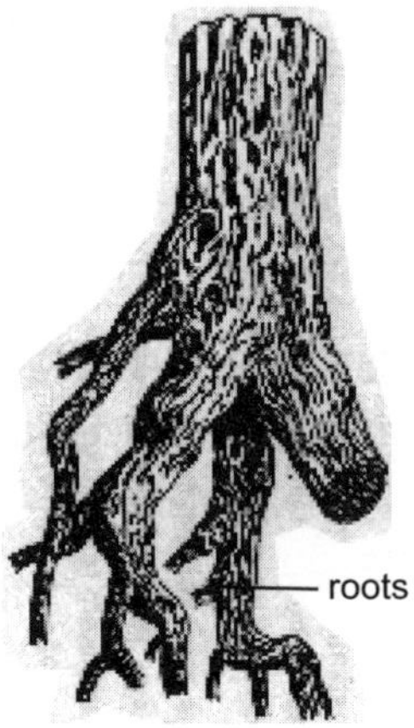

Fig. 7.3 Roots of Liquorice

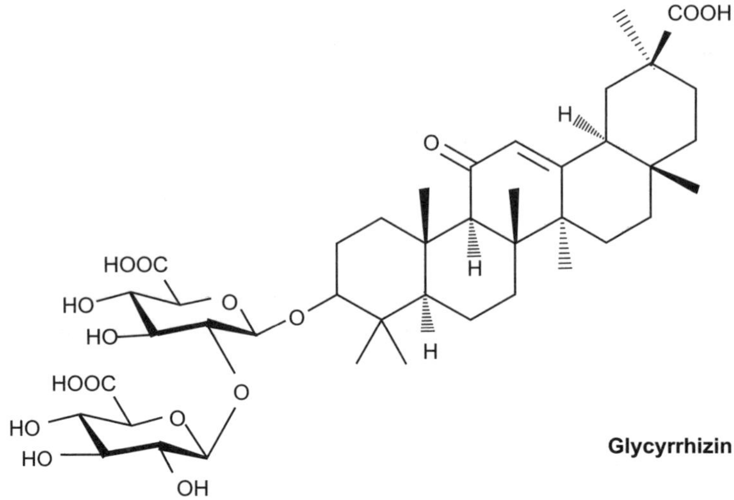

Glycyrrhizin

50 g of powdered drug is taken in a 500 ml beaker. 100 ml of methanol is added to mix and wet the sample. Another 100 ml of methanol is added and allowed to stand for 24 hours. This is then filtered and the filtrate is collected. This methanolic extract is extracted with three 5-ml portions of petroleum ether, subsequently with benzene (5 × 5 ml), ethyl acetate, chloroform and solvent ether. The methanolic layer is then transferred into a china dish and evaporated on a water bath to get glycyrrhizin.

Ammonium extraction method

The precipitate obtained by the first method is dissolved in dilute ammonium hydroxide (NH_4OH), followed by precipitation with the addition of acetone to obtain ammonium glycyrrhizinate.

Glycyrrhiza is extracted with hot water and filtered. The filtrate is acidified with concentrated H_2SO_4 to a pH of 2.8. The precipitate obtained is dissolved in dilute ammonium hydroxide and poured into acetone to precipitate ammonium glycyrrhizinate. The precipitate is dissolved in hot water and evaporated to get ammonium glycyrrhizinate.

TESTS FOR IDENTIFICATION

Foam test Being a saponin, glycyrrhizin produces froth (foam) in aqueous solution.

Salkowski test Chloroform solution of glycyrrhizin gives yellow colour on shaking with 1 ml of concentrated sulphuric acid.

Trichloroacetic acid test Chloroform solution of glycyrrhizin gives a deep red coloration with trichloroacetic acid.

TLC

Adsorbent	:	Kiesel gel 60 HF 254
Solvent system	:	Toluene, ethyl acetate and glacial acetic acid (12.5:7.5:0.5)
Reference standard	:	5 mg glycyrrhizin is refluxed with 20 ml of 0.5 ml H_2SO_4. On cooling, it is extracted with chloroform. When the chloroform extract is evaporated, the residue is dissolved in 1 ml of chloroform and methanol (1:1) mixture.
Test solution	:	1 g of the drug is shaken with 20 ml of chloroform and then filtered. The marc is refluxed with 30 ml of 0.5M H_2SO_4 for one hour. After cooling, the unfiltered mixture is extracted with chloroform. The extract is then concentrated and the residue is dissolved in 1 ml of chloroform and methanol (1:1) mixture.

Visualization

- Under UV light at 254 nm, the R_f value of 0.41 corresponds to glycyrrhetic acid in both test and standard reference samples.
- On spraying with anisaldehyde–sulphuric acid reagent, glycyrrhetic acid is visible as a dark violet spot in both samples.

ESTIMATION

TLC densitometric method

Adsorbent	:	Kiesel gel 60 HF 254
Solvent system	:	*n*-Butanol, acetic acid and water (7:1:2)
Detection	:	1% cerric sulphate in 10% H_2SO_4; heated at 105°C for 5 minutes.
Standard solution	:	Known concentration of glycyrrhizin (0.5–2.0 mg/ml) in 50% ethanol
Sample solution	:	1 g of the sample is refluxed with 50 ml of 50% ethanol. After cooling and filtration, the marc is refluxed again with 50 ml of 50% ethanol. On evaporation, the residue is dissolved in 50% ethanol (10 ml).
Development of chromatograms	:	13–14 cm apart, application of 10 μl standard and sample
Visualization	:	The sample is visualized and scanned in the densitometer. The area of the spots corresponding to glycyrrhetic acid are integrated. The percentage composition in the sample is calculated.

Colorimetric method

The basis for this method is that glycyrrhizin gives purple colour with anisaldehyde in the presence of H_2SO_4. The intensity of colour developed is proportionate to the amount of glycyrrhizin. The absorbance is measured at 556 nm.

UV spectroscopy

Glycyrrhizin forms a sodium salt with NaOH. In the procedure, sample and standards are weighed and dissolved in NaOH. The absorbance is measured at 258 nm. In another method, glycyrrhizin is dissolved in 80% ethanol and measured at 250 nm.

HPTLC method

Adsorbent	:	Silica gel GF 254
Mobile phase	:	Toluene, ethyl acetate and glacial acetic acid (12.5: 7.5: 0.5)
Detection	:	254 nm
Retention time	:	0.41 minutes

HPLC method

Column	:	Nova pack C18, reversed phase
Mobile phase	:	Acetonitrile, water and phosphoric acid (36:63:1)
Flow rate	:	1.4 ml/minute
Detection	:	UV at 250 nm
Standard	:	1 mg concentration. From this, serial dilutions containing 0.1, 0.2, 0.4, 0.6, 0.8 mg/ml in methanol are made.
Sample	:	1 g is extracted with water on the water bath, the extract is cooled and the volume is made up to 100 ml. 10 μl of standard and sample are injected separately into the HPLC column. The peak areas are recorded and, through the integrator, the amount is estimated.

7.6 GYMNEMIC ACID

It is a complex mixture of at least nine closely related acidic glycosides possessing anti-saccharine property. It is the active constituent of *Gymnema sylvestre* and other species of Gymnema. This plant is popularly known as Gur-mar ('destroyer of sugar').

Biological source

The leaves of *Gymnema sylvestre* belong to the Asclepiadaceae family.

Isolation

The dried powdered leaf is extracted with petroleum ether at 30°C–60°C. The marc is extracted with water and the aqueous extract is treated with 10% HCl to adjust the pH to 2. The precipitate that is obtained is centrifuged, washed with water and the dried residue containing crude gymnemic acid is divided into two portions.

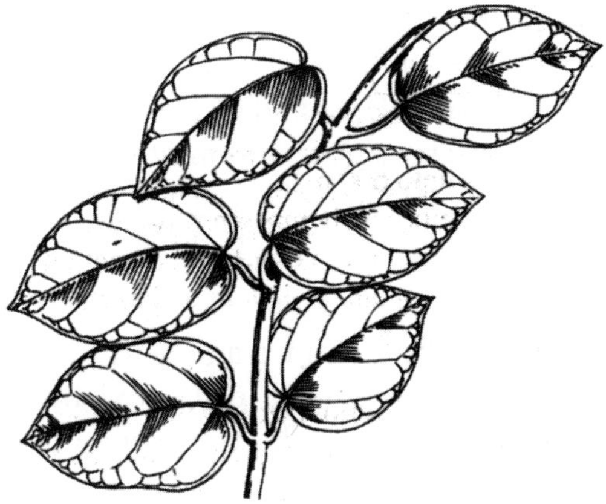

Fig. 7.4 Leaves of gymnema

The first portion is extracted with acetone in a mechanical shaker. The acetone extract containing the soluble acid is subjected to chromatography on silicic acid to obtain closely related gymnemic acids V to Z.

The second portion is plated on silicic acid and extracted with chloroform; the marc is further extracted with ethyl acetate. This ethyl acetate extract is then chromatographed on silicic acid to obtain the closely related gymnemic acids A to D.

Tests for identification

TLC

Adsorbent : Silica gel GF 254
Solvent system : Chloroform, isopropanol and ammonia (2:8:2)
Spray reagent : Anisaldehyde–sulphuric acid R_f: 0.45

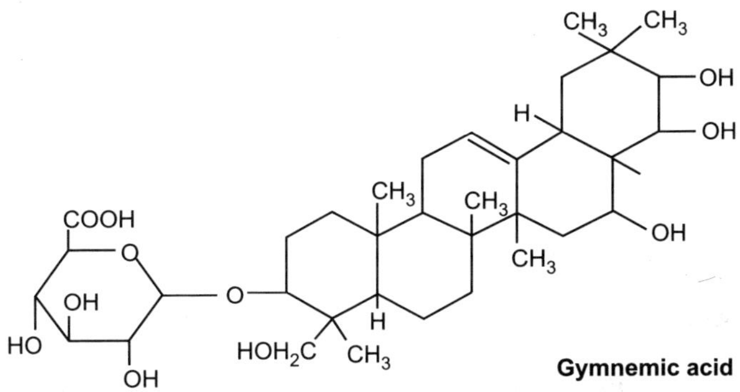

Gymnemic acid

Lieberman–Burchard reaction

Dissolve a small quantity of the isolated gymnemic acid in chloroform in a dry test tube. Add around 10 drops of acetic anhydride and 2 drops of concentrated H_2SO_4 and mix well. The colour of the solution changes from pink to green, indicating presence of an unsaturated steroid ring.

ESTIMATION

Crude gymnemic acid in the dry leaf extract and purified dry extract is estimated by gravimetry. Total gymnema saponin can be estimated by HPLC. In the procedure, gymnemagenin, which is the main sapogenin, is obtained by hydrolysis of a mixture of gymnemic acids.

Standard: Known concentration of 0.010 g of gymnemagenin in 100 ml of 50% ethanol.

Test sample: 0.75 g is dissolved in 50% ethanol. It is treated with 12% KOH by heating on a water bath for one hour. After cooling, 4N hydrochloric acid is added and heated for one hour. The pH is then adjusted to between 7.5 and 8.5 with 12% KOH. Finally, the volume is adjusted with 50% ethanol, filtered and subjected to HPLC.

HPLC column : Wakosil 5 C18, 4.6 mm × 25 cm
Gradient elution : Eluent A Acetonitrile and water (80:20)
Eluent B Potassium dihydrogen phosphate and water (0.1:100)
Flow rate : 1.5 ml/minute
UV detector : 210 nm
Standard and sample injection : 20 μl
Column temperature : 40°C

The peak heights are recorded and accordingly, the amount of gymnemic acid is estimated by considering the molecular weight of gymnemagenin and gymnemic acid II.

7.7 PHYLLANTHIN

Phyllanthin and hypophyllanthin are lignans. Phyllanthin is a diarlybutane whereas hypophyllanthin is an aryl tetrahydronaphthalein. They are the two major constituents of the plant *Phyllanthus amarus*.

BIOLOGICAL SOURCE

Aerial tender branches of *Phyllanthus amarus* belonging to Euphorbiaceae family are the main source of phyllanthin.

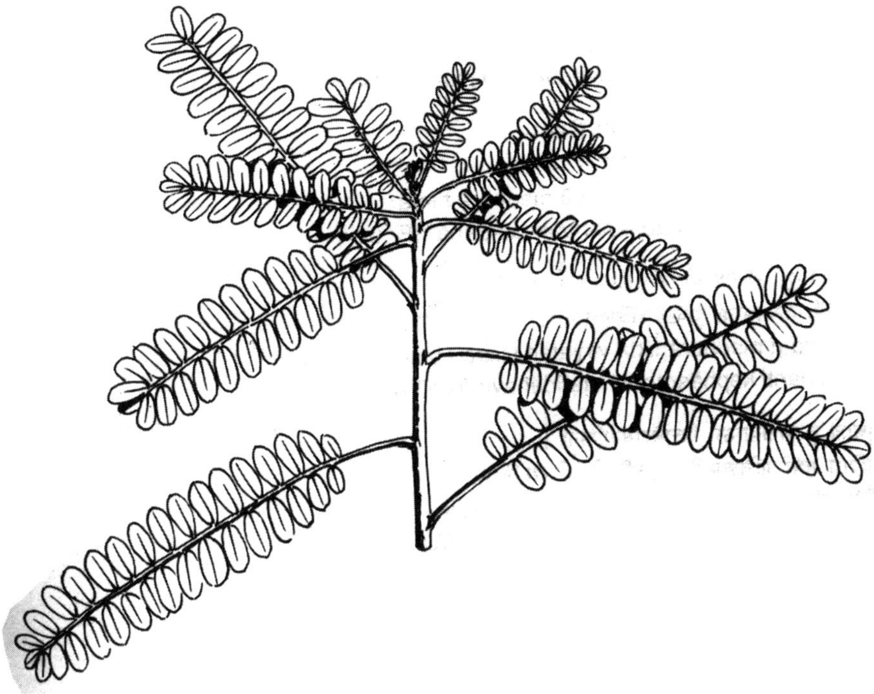

Fig. 7.5 Tender branches of Phyllanthus

Isolation

The powdered aerial parts of *Phyllanthus amarus* are mixed with lime and water, dried overnight and exhaustively extracted with petroleum ether in a Soxhlet extractor. The petroleum ether extract is then concentrated under reduced pressure and mixed with methanol by boiling. This procedure is repeated thrice and the de-waxed methanol extract is evaporated to dryness, and then dissolved in petroleum ether. This is next concentrated and allowed to stand to allow separation of the yellow oil. The residue obtained is fractionated by column chromatography on neutral alumina and eluted

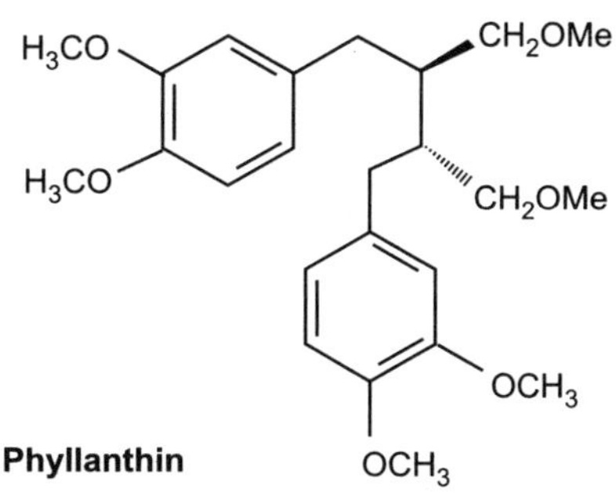

Phyllanthin

with *n*-hexane and ethyl acetate (99:1). The 99–108 fraction contains hypophyllanthin, whereas the 109–137 fraction contains phyllanthin as the major constituent. These fractions are further chromatographed to yield pure hypophyllanthin and phyllanthin.

Tests for identification

TLC is the main method with the following parameters.

Adsorbent	:	Silica gel GF 254
Solvent system	:	*n*-hexane and ethyl acetate (2:1)
Detection	:	Sulphuric acid reagent
R_f	:	Phyllanthin—0.20, blue spot Hypophyllanthin—0.25, brown spot

Estimation

HPLC is the main method of estimation.

Column	:	H-Bondapak C18
Mobile phase	:	Methanol and water (66:34)
Flow rate	:	1.8 ml/minute
Detection	:	UV at 230 nm
Standard	:	Known concentration in the range of 0.05–2 µg

Preparation of sample

1 g is macerated with lime and water at room temperature for 18 hours. It is then refluxed with 30 ml methanol containing 3% KOH for one hour. This is then cooled and filtered. The marc is again refluxed with methanol containing 3% KOH and filtered. This filtrate and the previous filtrate are combined and concentrated under reduced pressure and the volume is made up to 50 ml.

10 µl of standard and sample are injected separately into the HPLC column. The peak areas are recorded and the percentage concentration is calculated.

7.8 ASIATICOSIDE AND MADECASSOSIDE

Asiaticoside and madecassoside are the important triterpenoid saponins of mandukaparni or brahmi.

Biological source

The dried aerial parts, preferably the leaves of *Centella asiatica* belonging to the Apiaceae family, are the main source.

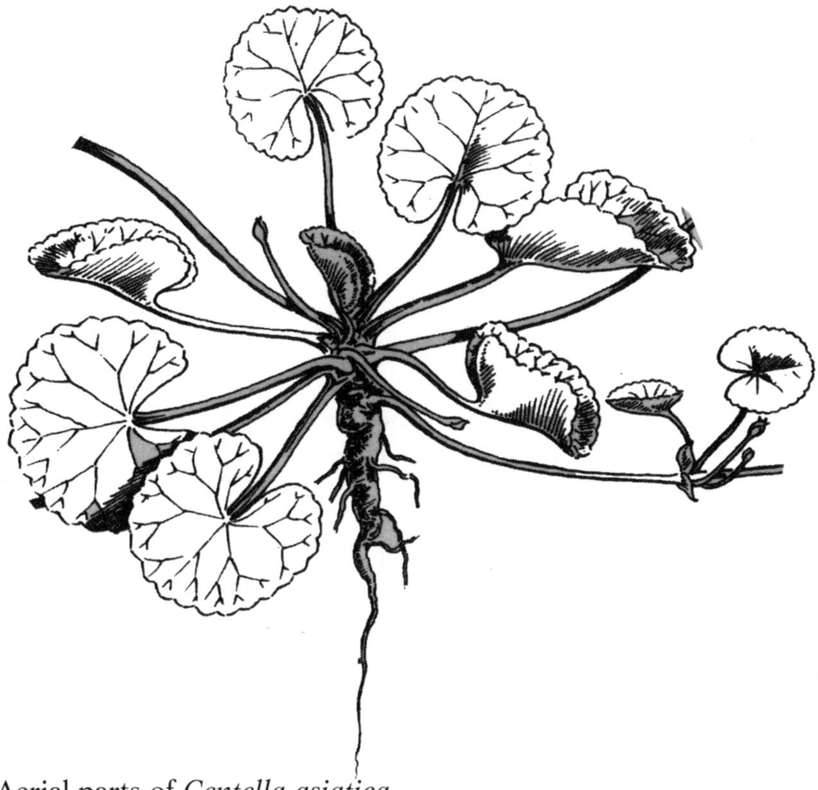

Fig. 7.6 Aerial parts of *Centella asiatica*

Isolation

The powdered whole plant is percolated with 90% alcohol. The alcohol extract is then subjected to partition chromatography by successive extractions with petroleum ether, diethyl ether, ethyl acetate and *n*-butanol. The *n*-butanol is recovered from the extract and the residue is extracted with three portions of acetone for one hour. This is then filtered while hot and the filtrate on cooling gives a cream coloured precipitate. It is then

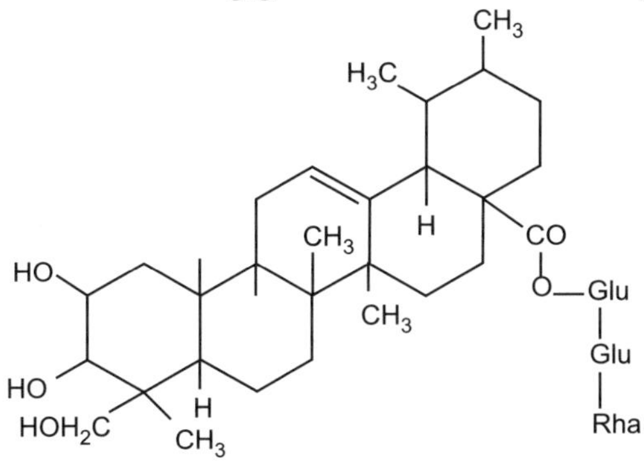

Asiaticoside

subjected to preparative HPLC with methanol and water (1:3), leading to the isolation of asiaticoside and madecassoside.

Tests for identification

Asiaticoside answers the tests for triterpenoid saponins: Salkowski test, Lieberman–Burchard reaction and trichloroacetic acid test.

Estimation

HPLC is used for estimation.

Column	:	μ-Bondapak C18 cartridge (8 mm × 10 cm)
Mobile phase	:	Acetonitrile and water (1:3)
Flow rate	:	1.5 ml/minute
Detection	:	UV at 205 nm
Standard	:	Known concentration of asiaticoside (0.02–0.4 mg/ml in methanol) and madecassoside (0.2–0.4 mg/ml)

Preparation of sample

2 g of the drug is refluxed with 90% methanol on a water bath. This is then cooled and filtered. The marc is then extracted again with 90% methanol and filtered. The two filtrates are combined and concentrated under vacuum. The volume is then made up to 50 ml and dilutions are made as per the requirement.

10 μl of standard and sample are injected separately into the HPLC column. The peak areas are recorded and the percentage of asiaticoside and madecassoside present in the sample is calculated.

7.9 ANDROGRAPHOLIDE

Andrographolide is the bitter principle (bioactive principle) of kalmegh. Chemically, it is a bicyclic diterpenoid lactone.

Biological source

Kalmegh consists of dried leaves and tender shoots of *Andrographis paniculata* belonging to Acanthaceae family.

Isolation

Andrographolide is soluble in methanol and ethanol; this property is used in the isolation of the active constituent. The dried powder of kalmegh is extracted successively with

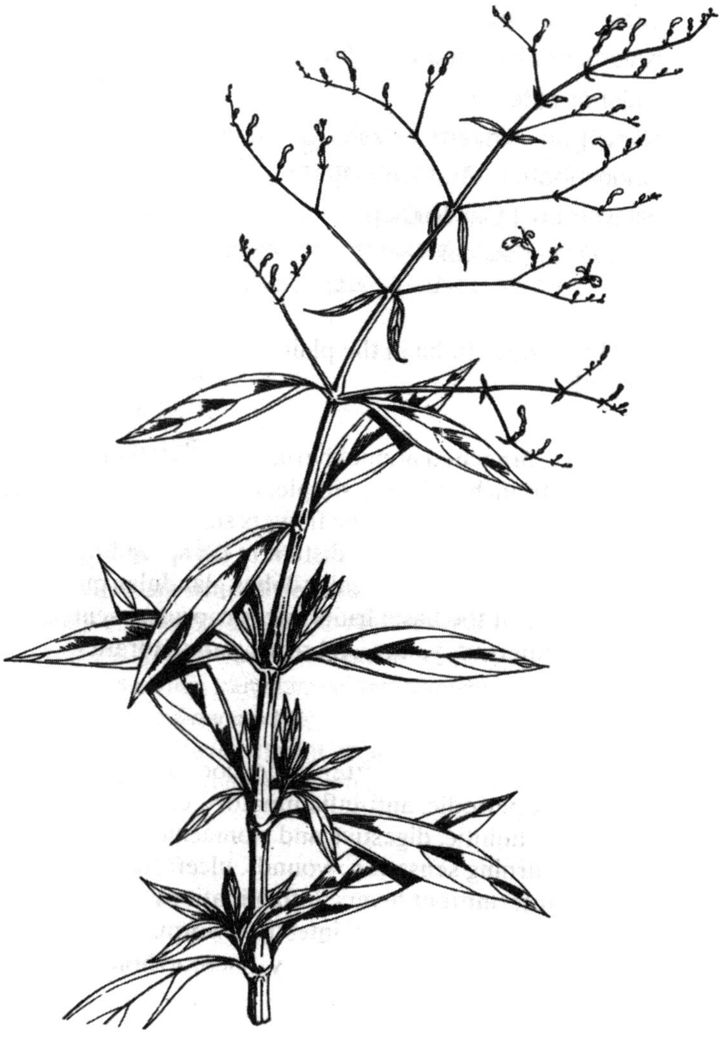

Fig. 7.7 Dried leaves of kalmegh

petroleum ether (60–80°C), chloroform and methanol. The methanolic extract is collected and concentrated. This is then treated with charcoal for 24 hours, filtered and the filtrate concentrated. This solution is kept overnight to crystallize and the crystals are collected by filtration. The recovered charcoal is next refluxed with methanol, filtered and the filtrate is added to the mother liquor. This is kept overnight for crystallization; the combined crystals are purified from methanol to get andrographolide with melting point of 228–229°C.

Tests for Identification

Copper acetate test

Since andrographolide is a diterpenoid it gives emerald green coloration.

TLC

Adsorbent	:	Silica gel 60 (precoated plates)
Solvent system	:	Chloroform and methanol (7:1)
Standard reference	:	Solution in methanol containing 1 mg/1.5 ml of methanol.
Sample solution	:	5 g of powdered drug is extracted with 50 ml of methanol. This methanolic extract is heated to obtain a residue. 10 mg of this residue is dissolved in 1 ml of methanol. 5 μl of standard and test solutions are used for spotting.
Development of chromatogram	:	15 cm Scanning at 223 nm for finger print profile and quantification
Visualization (post scanning)	:	Heated at 120°C for 10 minutes with 20% H_2SO_4 in methanol
R_f	:	0.7

Estimation

The common methods used are gravimetry, colorimetry and HPLC.

Colorimetry

Andrographolide gives red colour with alcoholic KOH which is measured at 400–800 nm.

HPLC method

Column	:	5 µm spherical silica
Mobile phase	:	Chloroform and methanol (9:1)
Flow rate	:	0.7•ml/minute
Detection	:	UV at 254 nm
Standard	:	Known concentration of andrographolide (0.5–10 mg/ml) in mobile phase.
Sample	:	The drug is extracted with methanol and evaporated. The residue is dissolved in methanol to give a strength of 50 µl/ml. 10 µl of standard and sample are injected separately into the HPLC column. The peak areas are recorded and the percentage of sample is estimated.

7.10 RUTIN

Chemically, it is quercetin-3-rutinoside. It is present up to 25% in any local flora. It is the most important and widespread of all the quercetin glycosides (about 200).

BIOLOGICAL SOURCE

Buckwheat : *Fagophyrum esculentum* (Polygonaceae)
Rhubarb : *Rheum emodi* (Polygonaceae)
Tobacco : *Nicotiana tabacum* (Solanaceae)
Rutea graveolens (Rutaceae)
Eucalyptus macroryncha (Myrtaceae)
Tea : *Thea sinensis* (Theaceae)

ISOLATION

20 g of powdered *Eucalyptus macroryncha* leaves are added to 500 ml of boiling water, and the mixture is boiled for 30 minutes. This is filtered while hot through several layers of cloth placed in a funnel. The filtrate is cooled for the precipitation of rutin. This is then filtered and re-crystallized from boiling water. This is again filtered and the rutin is collected on filter paper and allowed to dry.

TESTS FOR IDENTIFICATION

The main test is two-dimensional paper chromatography with the following parameters.

Solvent system : *n*-butanol, acetic acid, water and 5% acetic acid
Detection : visible, UV light
Standard reference : Rutin

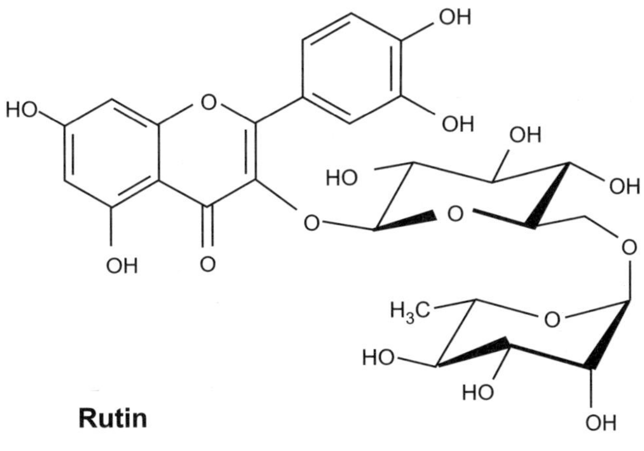

Rutin

Sample	:	powdered drug—70% alcohol extracted powdered drug extracted with 70% alcohol fresh drug; 90% alcohol extracted or fresh drug extracted with 90% alcohol
Estimation	:	Colorimetry
Standard solution	:	100 µg/ml of rutin in alcohol

Preparation of sample

A sample equivalent to 10 mg rutin is weighed and added to 80 ml of ethanol. The solution is boiled on a water bath and cooled to room temperature. The volume is made up to 100 ml with ethanol.

Composition	**Standard** (ml)	**Standard blank** (ml)	**Sample** (ml)	**Sample blank** (ml)
Prepared soln	2	2	2	2
Alc. $AlCl_3$	3	—	3	—
CH_3COOH	5	5	5	5
1N HCl	1	1	1	1
Distilled water	—	3	—	3

PROCEDURE The solution is allowed to stand at room temperature for 20 minutes. The volume is then made up to 25 ml. The absorbance of the sample is measured against the sample blank and that of the standard against the standard blank at 420 nm. The amount is calculated by comparison.

7.11 GUGGUL LIPIDS

BIOLOGICAL SOURCE

Guggul is the oleogum resin obtained by making deep incisions at the basal part of the stem bark of *Commiphora mukul* (*C. weightii*) belonging to family Burseraceae.

It is used as an anti-inflammatory, anti-rheumatic, hypocholesteremic drug. Guggul lipid is an anti-hyperlipidemic product of *C. mukul*. Guggul is an important ingredient of various ayurvedic formulations.

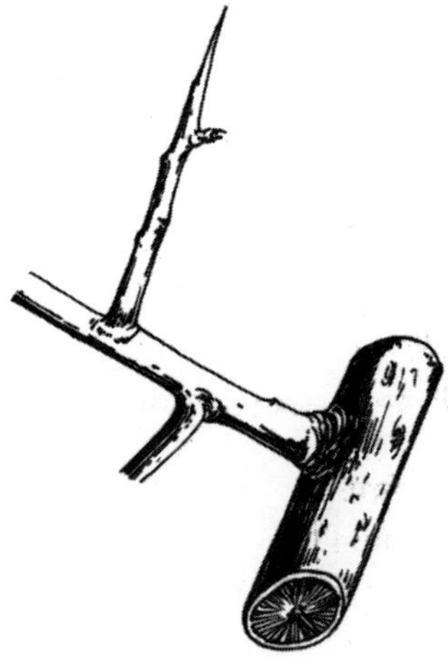

Fig. 7.8 Twig of guggul

EXTRACTION

The oleogum resin is extracted with ethyl acetate at 120–130°C. The insoluble portion is the gum, and the soluble portion consists of the oleoresin. Of this oleo-resin, the acidic portion has the anti-inflammatory component. The neutral portion is made up of ketonic and non-ketonic components. The ketonic part consists of Z-guggulsterone and E-guggulsterone; the latter having hypolipidaemic and hypocholesteremic actions.

PROCEDURE Guggul is extracted about 5 times with ethyl acetate. The extract is concentrated and the solvent is recovered. The oleo resin is purified by solvent fractionation for the enrichment of the guggulsterones. It is then thoroughly freed from the solvent under high vacuum. The guggul gum soft extract contains not less than 60% of guggul lipids and not less than 15% of guggulsterones.

ESTIMATION

Guggul lipids are estimated by isolation and weighing. About 2 g of the sample are extracted with three 20-ml portions of *n*-hexane with refluxing. After filtration, the filtrates are combined. The residue and filter paper are washed with 5 ml of *n*-hexane. The combined filtrates are evaporated in a tared beaker to dryness. This is then heated at 80°C for 1 hour under vacuum to a constant weight. The percentage of lipids can be calculated from the amount of sample.

Guggulsterones are estimated by spectrophotometry. A known amount of sample is refluxed with 0.5N alcoholic KOH and transferred to a separating funnel. The flask is washed with lukewarm water and the washings are added to the separating funnel. This is then extracted with three portions of petroleum ether. The petroleum ether extracts are then combined, the solvent is evaporated, and the residue is weighed. 0.1 g of the residue is taken and 10 ml of methanol is added. 1 ml of this solution is taken and diluted to 10 ml with methanol and the absorbance is measured at 327 nm, using methanol as a blank.

7.12 CARDIAC GLYCOSIDES

Cardiac glycosides exert highly specific and powerful actions on the cardiac muscle. They are used therapeutically to strengthen the heart and improve its efficiency. The aglycone part of these glycosides is the steroid moiety. Cardiac glycosides are classified as cardenolides (C23 glycosides) and bufadienolides (C24 glycosides).

Cardenolides contain a 5-membered α, β-unsaturated lactone at the 17th position which is of β-orientation. These glycosides are more prevalent in nature. The important drugs containing cardenolides are digitalis and strophanthus.

Bufadienolides contain a 6-membered doubly unsaturated lactone at the 17th position. Squill is an example of this class.

CARDIAC GLYCOSIDES OF *DIGITALIS PURPUREA*

The main glycosides of *Digitalis purpurea* include purpurea glycoside A (PGA), purpurea glycoside B (PGB) and glucogitaloxin. They are tetrasides. On enzymatic hydrolysis, the following triosides are formed:

PGA ⟶ Digitoxin and glucose
PGB ⟶ Gitoxin and glucose
Glucogitaloxin ⟶ Gitaloxin and glucose

Digitoxin is the primary active constituent of *D. purpurea*. Digitoxigenin, gitoxigenin and gitaloxigenin are the aglycones of digitoxin, gitoxin and gitaloxin respectively, which are formed by acid hydrolysis. *D. purpurea* also contains a number of cardenolides including biosides and monosides.

ISOLATION

Modified Stas Otto procedure can be followed for the extraction of cardiac glycosides from *D. purpurea* and *D. lanata*. Two methods are available and the selection of the method depends on the nature of the material, i.e., whether it is fresh or dry.

Extraction from dried material
Enzymes are inactive in the dried material. The coarse powdered drug is macerated with 70% alcohol for 1 hour. It is filtered and the filtrate is treated with a strong solution of lead acetate to precipitate pigments, proteins and alkaloidal substances. The supernatant liquid is collected on centrifugation. Excess lead is precipitated with 6.3% Na_2SO_4 solution. It is further centrifuged and the supernatant liquid is collected. This is then extracted with three portions of chloroform. The combined extract is then evaporated for the crystallization of glycosides.

Extraction from fresh leaves
In this method prior deactivation of enzyme is required. The fresh drug is homogenized with water and heated at 70°C for deactivating the enzymes and coagulation of proteins. The supernatant liquid collected on centrifugation is treated with anhydrous sodium sulphate (Na_2SO_4) to saturate the solution. The glycosides are absorbed on kieselguhr to form colloidal glycoside precipitate. This is then collected by filtration on Buchner funnel. Filtration is continued till the residue is dry. Finally, the dried residue is extracted with methylethyl ketone.

ISOLATION OF DIGITOXIN

The powdered drug is macerated with water at 45°C for 4–5 hours and the aqueous extract is collected. The marc is macerated with 20% methanol for 24 hours and the

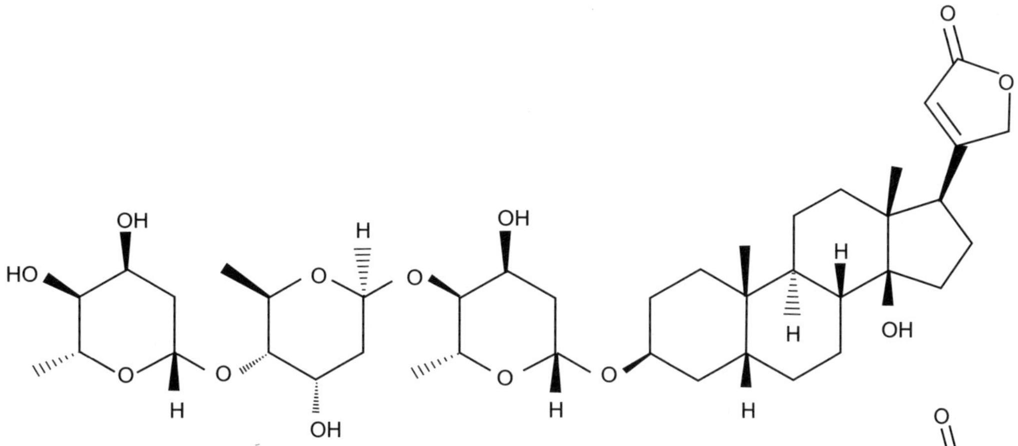

Digitoxin

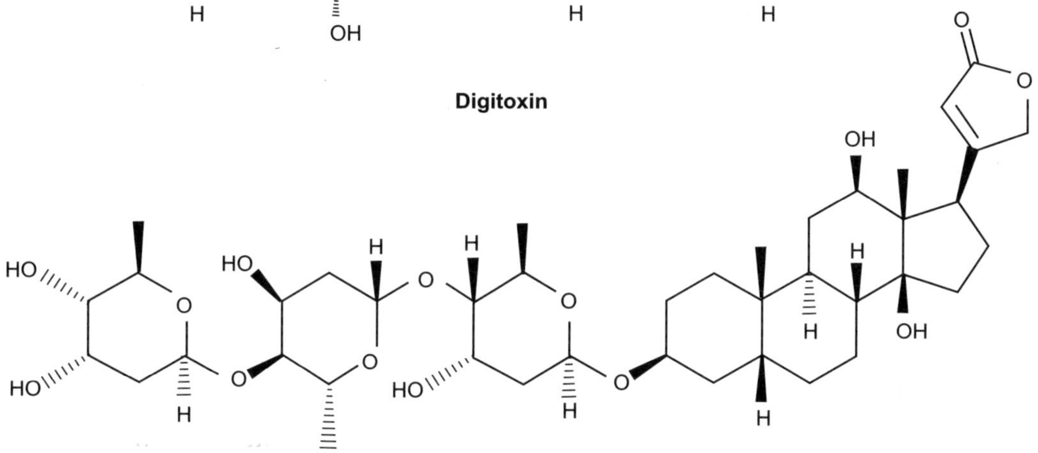

Digoxin

methanolic extracts are collected. The aqueous and methanolic extracts are combined and made alkaline with NaOH so as to cause hydrolysis. This is then extracted with chloroform and evaporated to dryness. The residue obtained is subjected to column chromatography with the following parameters:

Adsorbent : Silica gel G
Solvent system : Gradient elution initially with carbon tetrachloride followed by ethyl acetate and methanol.

The carbon tetrachloride fraction contains colouring matter (pigments), the ethyl acetate fraction has flavones and anthraquinones, whereas the methanolic fraction contains digitoxin with R_f value of 0.486. Digitoxin is purified by re-crystallization from alcohol and diethyl ether (1:1) mixture.

TESTS FOR IDENTIFICATION

The general chemical tests for cardiac glycosides are listed on next page.

Legal test

The drug extract is dissolved in pyridine and sodium nitroprusside solution is added. A yellow to orange colour is obtained on making the solution alkaline.

Baljet test

The sample gives pink to red coloration with sodium picrate.

Keller–Killiani test

The powdered drug is extracted by heating with 70% alcohol, the extract is filtered. The filtrate is mixed with water; a strong solution of lead acetate is added and shaken. This is again filtered, and the filtrate is mixed with an equal volume of chloroform. The chloroform layer is collected and evaporated; the residue obtained is dissolved in glacial acetic acid, cooled and two drops of ferric chloride are added. This is transferred to a test tube containing 2 ml of concentrated H_2SO_4 to obtain a reddish brown layer that slowly turns to bluish green.

Kedde's test

The sample is treated with 3, 5-dinitrobenzoic acid in methanol and KOH solution to give a reddish or bluish violet colour.

Raymond's test

The sample gives a bluish violet coloration with dinitrobenzene and methanolic potassium hydroxide.

Estimation

Spectroscopy, bioassay and HPLC are the main methods of estimation.

Spectroscopy

Cardenolides can be estimated by the measurement of absorbance based on the digitoxose moiety and lactone ring. The digitoxose moiety reacts in the Keller–Killiani test to form a product that shows λ_{max} of 590 nm. The lactone ring on reaction with *m*-dinitrobenzene gives a product with λ_{max} of 620 nm.

IP method for estimation of digitoxin

About 40 mg of digitoxin is weighed and dissolved in 100 ml of ethanol. 5 ml of this solution is diluted to 100 ml with ethanol. 3 ml of alkaline picric acid solution is added to 5 ml of the diluted solution and allowed to stand for 30 minutes. The absorbance is measured against a blank at 495 nm.

Bioassay

Digitalis and its preparations can be biologically assayed for their potency. The IP suggests the use of both pigeons and guinea pigs as test animals. Comparison of the effect of a known dilution of the drug with that of the similar dilution of standard preparation forms the basis of bioassay. Adult pigeons are anaesthetized lightly with ether. The vein of the immobilized pigeon is exposed and cannulated. Definite volumes of diluted preparations are introduced at 5 minute intervals until it dies from cardiac arrest. In the case of guinea pigs, the drug is administered into the jugular vein.

HPLC method

The following parameters are used for estimation of *D. purpurea* glycosides.

Column	:	Octyl silicyl bonded silica
Solvent system	:	Methyl cyanate, methyl alcohol and water (10:15:18)
Flow rate	:	0.5 ml/min
Detection wavelength	:	220 nm

Sample preparation About 50 mg of leaf powder is mixed with 50% methanol (25 ml) containing a known amount of lanatoside A as internal standard. This is subjected to ultrasonification for 1 hour, filtered and the filtrate is evaporated to dryness in vacuum. The residue is dissolved in 2 ml of a mixture of methyl cyanate and water (1:9) and subjected to column chromatography, eluting with a 1:1 mixture of methyl cyanate and water. This eluate is dried and dissolved in 1 ml of mobile phase.

Method 10 μl of the sample is subjected to HPLC. The peak areas of purpurea glycoside A, B, glucogitaloxin, digitoxin, gitoxin and gitaloxin are recorded and their amounts can be estimated by their peak area ratios with the internal standard.

7.13 ATROPINE

Atropine is a tropane alkaloid obtained from the members of the Solanaceae family. It is present in *Atropa belladonna*, *Datura stramonium*, and *Hyoscyamus niger*. Other important solanaceous alkaloids are hyoscyamine, hyoscine, apoatropine, belladonnine and norhyoscyamine.

Isolation

Atropine is isolated from the juice or the powder drug of *Hyoscyamus muticus* which has the highest alkaloid content, followed by *Datura stramonium*. The drug material is powdered and wetted with an aqueous solution of sodium carbonate and then extracted with ether or benzene. The alkaloidal free bases are extracted from the solvent using water that has been acidified with acetic acid. Coloring matter is removed by shaking the acid solution with solvent ether. The alkaloids are precipitated using sodium carbonate, filtered, washed and dried. The dried mass is dissolved in solvent ether or acetone and dehydrated with

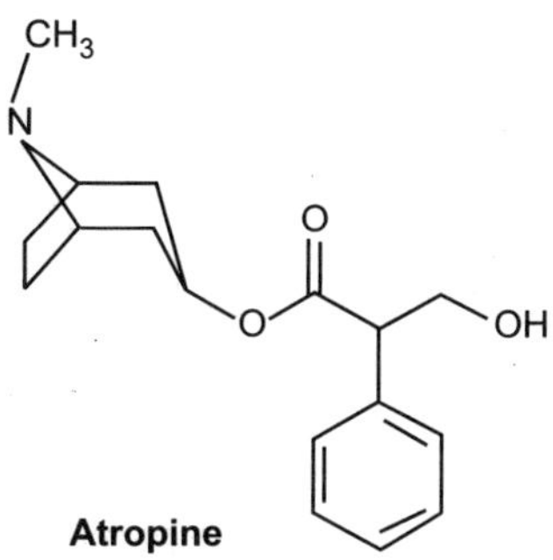

Atropine

anhydrous sodium sulphate. This is then filtered and the filtrate is concentrated and cooled to yield crude crystals of hyoscyamine and atropine from solution. The crude crystalline mass is separated from the solution and then dissolved in alcohol. Sodium hydroxide solution is added and the mixture is kept till hyoscyamine is completely racemised to atropine. This is indicated by the loss of optical activity. The crude atropine is purified by crystallization from acetone. Atropine sulphate, the most important salt of atropine, occurs in the form of a colourless, crystalline powder which is soluble in water and alcohol and insoluble in ether and chloroform.

Tests for identification

TLC

A 1% solution of atropine dissolved in 2N acetic acid is spotted over silica gel G plate and eluted in the solvent system of strong ammonia solution and methanol in a ratio of 1.5:100. TLC plate is spread with an acidified iodoplatinate solution. R_f value of atropine is 0.18.

Vitali–Mortein test

A dilute solution of atropine is treated with concentrated nitric acid and the mixture is evaporated to dryness on a steam bath. This produces a pale yellow residue which gives a violet colour with a solution of KOH.

7.14 VINCA ALKALOIDS

Vinblastine and vincristine are the two important vinca alkaloids used in the treatment of cancer. Vinblastine sulphate is useful in Hodgkin's disease and various neoplasms whereas vincristine is used in the treatment of sarcomas and acute hemocytic leukemia.

Biological source

It is the dried whole plant of *Catharanthus roseus* belonging to family Apocyanaceae (Madagascar periwinkle). The vinca alkaloids contian indole and dihydroindole units.

Isolation

Vinca leaves and herbs are minced and extracted with aqueous alcoholic acetic acid (CH_3COOH) solution. After concentration of the aqueous extract, the residue is further extracted with 2% HCl. NaOH is used to adjust the pH of the extract to 4. This is again extracted with benzene. The pH of the aqueous solution is then raised to 7 and again extracted with benzene. The pH-7 benzene extracts are mixed together, concentrated,

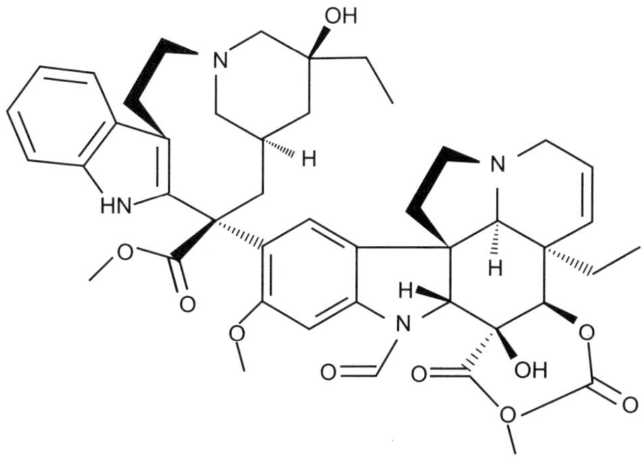

Vincristine

dried and dissolved in benzene–methylene chloride (65:35) solution. This is separated by chromatography on a neutral alumina column with benzene–methylene chloride solution as an eluent using gradient elution technique. Evaporation of the vinblastine-rich fractions gives vinblastine sulphate which is recrystallized from alcohol. Further elution of the column gives vincristine which is dried and crystallized from methanol.

Tests for identification

TLC is an efficient means to identify vinca alkaloids. 1 mg of sample alkaloid is dissolved in 0.1 ml of 25% water in methanol and spotted on silica gel G plate. The solvent system used is acetonitrile and benzene (30:70). Eluted plates are dried, sprayed with 1% solution of cerric ammonium sulphate in 85% phosphoric acid. Vincristine-free base gives R_f value of 0.39.

7.15 SOLASODINE

Solasodine is an aglycone of steroidal glycoalkaloid found in many species of solanaceous family.

Biological source

The various sources include *Solanum incanum, Solanum khasianum* and *Solanum xanthocarpum*. Solasonine is a steroidal alkaloid which yields the aglycone solasodine and sugars like mannose, glucose and galactose.

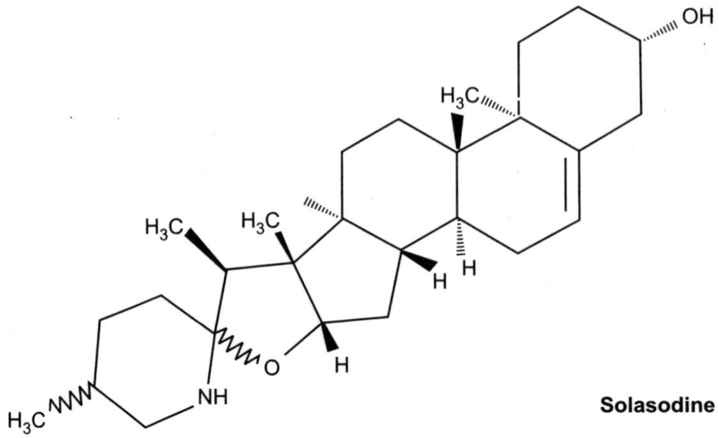

Solasodine

Isolation

The dried berries are first powdered and processed to remove fats using petroleum ether to give a greenish yellow oil; this is rejected. The de-fatted material is extracted three times using ethanol. The combined extracts are concentrated to one-tenth of the volume. Concentrated HCl is added and the solution is refluxed for about six hours to allow complete hydrolysis of the glycoalkaloid. The mixture is then made alkaline by adding ammonia and refluxed for one hour. The reaction mixture is cooled and filtered and the residue obtained is thoroughly washed with water till the pH becomes neutral; it is dried. The dried material is dissolved in chloroform, whereby solasodine moves into the chloroform layer. The solution is filtered and the solvent is evaporated to yield a residue containing solasodine. It is further purified by crystallizing from methanol.

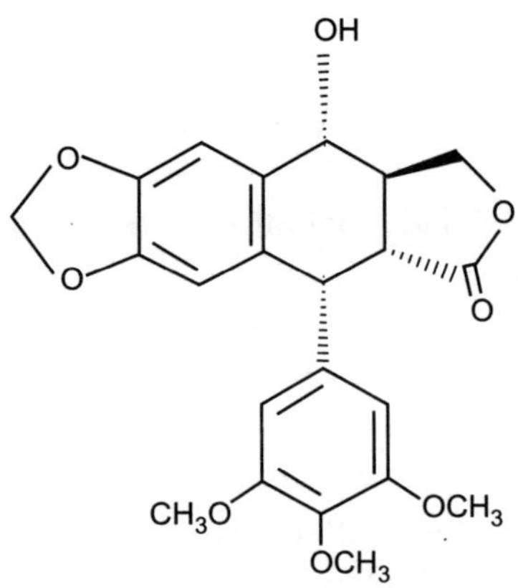

Podophyllotoxin

TESTS FOR IDENTIFICATION

1 mg of the sample and standard is dissolved in 1 ml of methanol separately. The test solution and standard solution are applied on silica gel G plates and developed in a solvent system containing toluene, ethyl acetate and diethylamine (7:2:1). The dried plates are sprayed with modified Dragendroff's reagent. The plate is allowed to dry and sprayed again with 10% sulphuric acid in methanol. Orange to red spots are seen. R_f value of solasodine is 0.60.

7.16 PODOPHYLLOTOXIN

Chemically, podophyllotoxin is a lignin compound with a 4-phenyl-tetrahydronapthalene-3-carboxylic acid lactone skeleton. It is used widely as an anti-rheumatic, anti-viral and anti-tumour agent.

BIOLOGICAL SOURCE

It is obtained from the dried rhizomes and roots of the American mandrake, *Podophyllum peltatum,* and also from Indian podophyllum, *P. hexandrum,* belonging to the family Berberidaceae.

ISOLATION

Podophyllum resin is extracted from dried rhizomes and roots using an alcoholic percolation method and subsequent precipitation from the concentrated percolate by adding acidified water. It contains not less than 40% of podophyllum resin and not more than 50% of hexane-insoluble matter.

The powdered and dried rhizomes and roots of podophyllum are extracted with 90% ethanol in a Soxhlet extractor. Alcohol is removed by distillation and the alcoholic extract is concentrated till it attains a syrup-like consistency. A mixture of water containing 2% HCl is poured into this syrup at 5°C with continuous stirring. The mixture is allowed to stand for two hours below 5°C and then filtered under vacuum. The residue is washed with acidified water, cooled below 5°C and then dissolved in sufficient quantity of 90% hot alcohol. This solution is filtered and the alcohol distilled off. The residue is further dried at 80°C to a constant weight.

TEST FOR IDENTIFICATION

Dissolve podophyllum resin and podophyllotoxin separately in methanol. Apply the spots over silica gel G plate and elute it first with chloroform and methanol (90:10) to a distance of 6 cm. At the end of this procedure, only the glycosides get separated, but the aglycone podophyllotoxin remains near the solvent front.The same TLC plate is again eluted with more weakly polar solvent chloroform and acetone (65:35), this time upto a distance of 12 cm. During the second stage of elution, the glycosides do not migrate but the aglycone moves. The dried plate is sprayed with H_2SO_4–acetic anhydride mixture (1:3), followed by heating at 100°C for 15 minutes. The zones and spots of glycosides and aglycone correspond to their standards. Podophyllotoxin gives a R_f value 0.65.

7.14 MENTHOL

Menthol is a monoterpene alcohol obtained from diverse types of mint oils or peppermint. Along with menthol, the oil contains (+) neomenthol, (+) isomenthol, menthone, menthofuran, menthyl acetate and cineol. The menthol obtained from natural sources is levorotatory (l-menthol) or racemic (dl-menthol).

Menthol

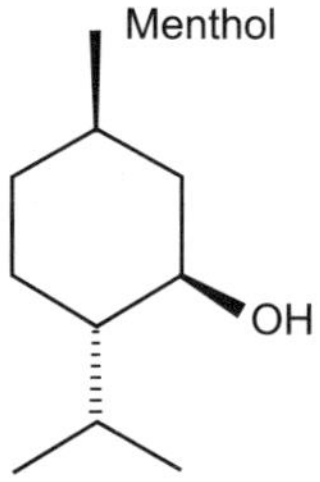

Biological source

The sources of mint oil include black peppermint *Mentha piperita* Var *vulgaris*; white peppermint *Mentha piperita* Var *officinalis*, *Mentha arvensis* and *Mentha canadensis* belonging to family Lamiaceae.

Isolation

Mentha oil is obtained from the hydrodistillation or steam distillation of fresh plant parts located above the soil just before flowering. For (–) menthol isolation from peppermint oil, the oil is subjected to cooling. The crystals of menthol crystallize out from the oil which can be separated by centrifugation.

Corn mint oil obtained from the steam distillation of the flowering herb *Mentha arvensis* contains about 70%–80% of free (–) menthol. Corn mint oil is cooled and the crystals of menthol produced are separated by centrifugation. Since the crystalline product contains traces of corn mint oil, this menthol has a slightly herbaceous mint-like flavour. Pure (–) menthol is obtained by recrystallization from solvents with low boiling points. Dementholized corn mint oil from which (–) menthol is removed by crystallization and which still contains 40%–50% free menthol can also be reused for producing (–) menthol.

Tests for identification

About 1 mg of menthol is dissolved in about 1 ml of methanol. The spot is applied on silica gel G plate and eluted in pure chloroform. The dried plates are sprayed with 1% vanillin–sulphuric acid reagent and heated at 110°C for 10 minutes. Menthol gives an R_f value of 0.48–0.62 when the chamber is saturated at 24°C.

7.18 CITRIC ACID

Citric acid is an organic acid which acts as a natural preservative and provides an acidic or sour taste to food and soft drinks. It exists naturally in various fruits and vegetables, but maximum concentrations are found in lemons and limes, where it makes up to about 8% of the dry weight of the fruit.

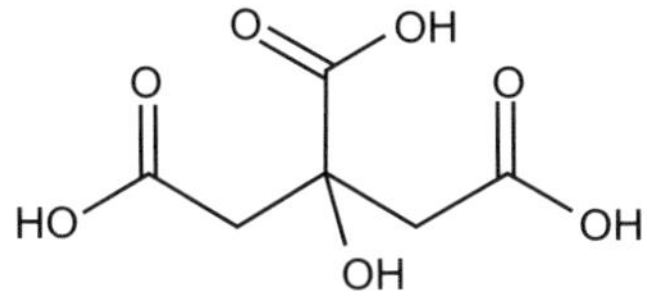

Citric acid

ISOLATION

The juice is squeezed out from lemon fruits and is made alkaline by adding 20% NaOH or KOH solution with continuous stirring. The change in pH can be identified by a change in the colour of the solution from yellow to pale brown. The solution is filtered using a Buchner funnel to remove all extraneous matter such as seeds and pulp. The filtrate is mixed with 10%–15% $CaCl_2$ solution and stirred well. The precipitate of calcium citrate obtained is separated by filtration and washed with boiling water.

Exercises

Long answers

1. Describe the process of isolation of calcium sennosides.
2. Discuss the method of isolation of ephedrine.
3. Explain in detail the various methods of estimation of ephedrine.
4. What are the methods for estimation of phyllanthin and rutin?
5. How is andrographolide isolated? Discuss any one method of estimating it.

Short answers

6. Explain the process of isolation of quinine from cinchona bark.
7. Describe the process of isolation of glycyrrhizin.
8. What are the tests for identification of digitalis glycosides?
9. Discuss the identification tests for asiaticoside.
10. Explain how menthol is isolated.

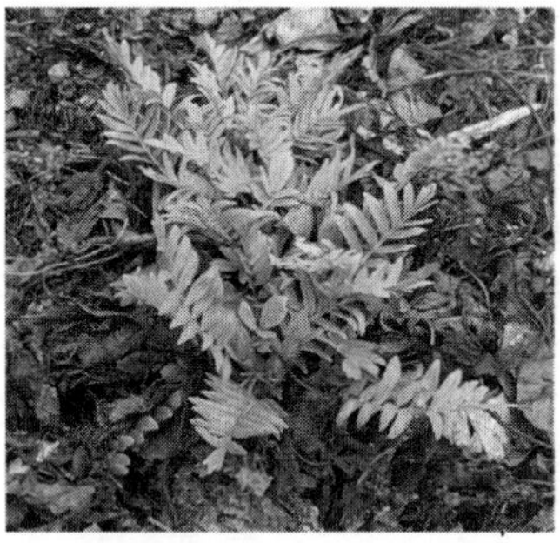

8

Herbal Cosmetics

In This Chapter, You Will Learn

- The functions of cosmetics
- Herbal cosmetics used in the care of skin and hair
- Biological source, family, chemical constituents and uses of some herbal cosmetics

Natural ingredients have been used in personal and health care products for many centuries. Modern research proves that herbs are effective and also mild and soothing. Potent synthetic preparations and chemicals though effective, constitute a toxic burden on the human body. Herbal cosmetics are mild and effective. Moreover, they are inexpensive and easily available. The most common application of herbs in cosmetics is in the preparation of skin and hair care cosmetics as well as dentifrices.

Various ingredients used in cosmetics are derived from plant parts. These include dried plant materials in powder form, pure compounds isolated from plants, fresh herbs, galenicals, unorganized drugs such as resins, gums, essential oils and fixed oils and certain standardized extracts with a known concentration of actives.

Herbal cosmetics

Herbal cosmetics are defined as beauty products obtained from natural sources with desirable physiological activities such as skin healing, smoothening, and appearance-enhancing and conditioning properties.

Herbal cosmetics contain products that can repair, revitalize and protect the skin, and prevent hair fall and promote hair growth. Perfumes, soaps and powders used for protective and cleansing action are also cosmetics.

Cosmetics have many uses.

- They are used in personal care products to keep the body clean and odour-free.
- They are used as perfumes in the form of oils and extracts.
- They are used to enhance appearance and thereby improve self-esteem.

Perfumes

Both vegetable- and animal-based perfumes are used in the preparation of herbal cosmetics. Vegetable perfumes contain essential oils with a pleasant fragrance. Rosemary oil, lavender oil and jasmine oil are widely used in cosmetic preparations. Various terpeneless essential oils are also used in herbal cosmetics. These oils are obtained by a process of distillation of crude oil to separate non-volatile materials or by adsorbtion of volatile components to provide the oxygenated constituents.

Animal perfumes mainly contain musk from the musk deer, which is used in preparing shaving creams, after-shave lotions and talcum powders. The special feature of this perfume is its ability to retain fragrance even after dilution by a factor of 3000. Civet is a perfume obtained from civet cats. It is procured from the specialized secretory glands in both female and male civet cats. Ambergris is a perfume obtained from the small intestine of the rare sperm whale.

Hair care

Several herbs have been used as hair growth promoters, revitalizers, conditioners, colouring agents and rinses. Some important preparations are oils, shampoos, hair tonics, conditioners and anti-dandruff agents.

Hair tonics and conditioners

They are used as part of daily care. Table 8.1 lists the herbs used as hair tonics and conditioners.

Table 8.1 Herbs used as hair tonics and conditioners

Herb	Used for
Amla	Conditioning, darkening and promoting hair growth
Henna	Conditioning, darkening and also promoting hair growth
Aloe vera gel	Conditioning hair
Jatamansi	Strengthening hair and reducing hair loss
Brahmi	Hair growth and cooling effect
Castor oil	Promoting hair growth (because it contains vitamin E)
Almond oil	Conditioning and hair dressing
Hibiscus	Conditioning hair
Rosemary oil	Keeping hair silky and fragrant
Bhringaraj	Promoting hair growth
Tea	Conditioning and darkening hair

Shampoos and hair rinses

Jaswand (*Hibiscus rosasinensis*), amla, bhringaraj (*Eclipta alba*), shikakai (*Acacia conccinna*), soapnut (*Sapindius trifoliatus*) and chamomile are used in shampoos and hair rinses.

Anti-dandruff agents

Rosemary oil, sandalwood oil and apricot have anti-dandruff properties.

Hair colour

Amla, henna, chamomile and tea decoctions give good colour and shine to the hair.

Skin care

Herbs are used in the preparation of skin care preparations to provide antiseptic, emollient, astringent, protective, and anti-ageing effects. Some of the herbs and their uses are listed below.

- *Turmeric* is a well-known antiseptic and anti-inflammatory agent.
- *Aloe vera gel* is an excellent emollient and moisturizer which smoothens rough skin and relieves skin irritation. It is commonly used in preparing sun tan lotions, soaps, shaving creams and baby oils.
- *Wheat germ oil* is obtained from the endosperm of wheat and is a by-product in the manufacture of starch from wheat. It has powerful antioxidant properties because it is rich in vitamin E and helps in softening the skin and improving its tone. It protects the skin against damage by ultraviolet radiation.
- *Neem* has strong and effective antiseptic action and is a common ingredient of soaps and creams.
- *Honey* is an excellent emollient.
- *Grapes* contain α-hydroxy amino acids (AHA), and in combination with aloe vera, make a good anti-wrinkle agent.
- *Almond oil, lanolin* and *apricot* are included in anti-wrinkle preparations.
- *Cucumber, papaya, orange peel, lemon peel* and *almond* have skin cleansing action.
- *Turmeric, aloe* and *galangal* are used for their bleaching action on the skin.

Dentifrices and herbal shampoos

Herbs such as babul (*Acacia arabica*), clove oil, peppermint oil, *Acacia catechu* and wintergreen oil are commonly used in the preparation of dentifrices such as toothpaste and tooth powder.

A shampoo is a liquid or gel used for washing the hair in order to clean, remove dandruff and give nourishment. Shampoo ingredients obtained from herbs include detergents such as soap bark, perfumes such as sandalwood oil, lemon and orange peel and cardamom oil. Shikakai, lavender, amla, hibiscus and lemon grass are used as conditioners. Ingredients such as tea tree oil and valerian are often included for their anti-dandruff action, whereas chamomile and neem have a deep cleansing action.

Some common herbal ingredients in cosmetics such as, soapnut, amla, henna, aloe vera, turmeric and sandal wood oil are discussed below.

8.1 SOAPNUT

BIOLOGICAL SOURCE

It is obtained from the dried ripe fruits of *Sapindus trifoliatus, Sapindus laurifolius* or *Sapindus emarginatus* belonging to the family Sapindaceae.

CHEMICAL CONSTITUENTS

It consists of 11.5 % saponins, 10% glucose and saponin glycosides. Emarginatoside is the most important saponin glycoside isolated from the aqueous extract of the fruit. On hydrolysis, this glycoside yields a sapogenin called hederagenin — (3β, 4α)-3, 23-dihydroxyolean-12-en-28-oic acid—D glucose, D xylose and L rhamnose. A cyclic sesquiterpene oligoglycoside called trifolioside has been recently isolated from the pericarp of the fruit. The kernels have 45% fixed oil containing palmitic, stearic, oleic, linoleic and arachidic acids.

USES

The pericarp of the fruit is used for its detergent action in the preparation of soaps and shampoos. Since saponins have a foaming action, they are effective in hair cleansing. These saponins are also used as excipients to prepare a vaccine against foot and mouth disease virus in guinea pigs.

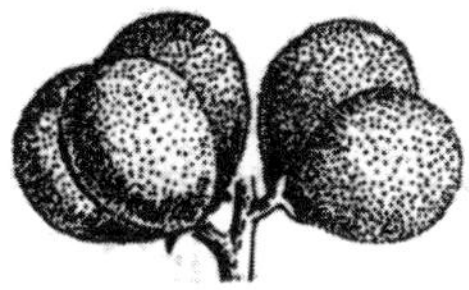

Fig. 8.1 Fruits of soapnut

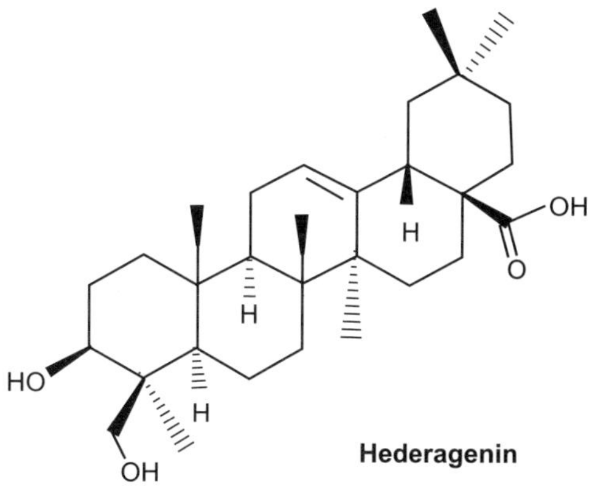

Hederagenin

Pessaries prepared from the kernels are often used as a uterine stimulant to aid in the process of childbirth. The roots and bark of the tree are used as a mild expectorant and demulscent. The fruits and bark also have a toxic action on fish and are therefore used as fish poison.

8.2 AMLA

Biological source

The main source is the fresh and dried fruit of *Emblica officinalis* (*Phyllanthus emblica*) belonging to the Euphorbiaceae family.

Chemical constituents

Amla is the richest natural source of vitamin C. It contains 500–950 mg vitamin C per 100 g of fresh pulp. Amla mainly contains tannins such as gallic acid, trigalloyl glucose, terchebin, corilegin, ellagic acid, phyllembic acid and emblicon. Alkaloids such as phyllantigine and phyllantine are also found. The immature fruits of amla have been found to contain indole acetic acid and the four auxins A1, A3, A4 and A5, besides two growth inhibitors, R1 and R2. The fruit is also a relatively rich source of pectin, and minerals such as calcium, phosphorous and iron.

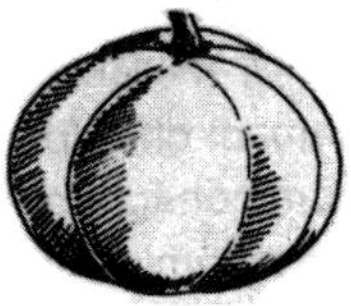

Fig. 8.2 Fruit of amla

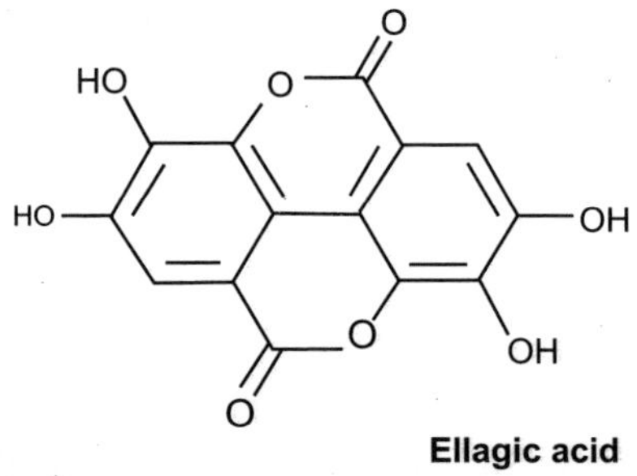

Ellagic acid

Uses

Traditionally, amla has been used in herbal cosmetics. Even today, it is a common ingredient in preparations such as hair conditioners and dyes, and in the treatment of dandruff. Amla also has significant anti-fungal, anti-bacterial, anti-viral and anti-oxidant properties.

8.3 HENNA

Biological source

Henna is obtained from the dried leaves of *Lawsonia inermis* or *Lawsonia alba* belonging to the Lythraceae family.

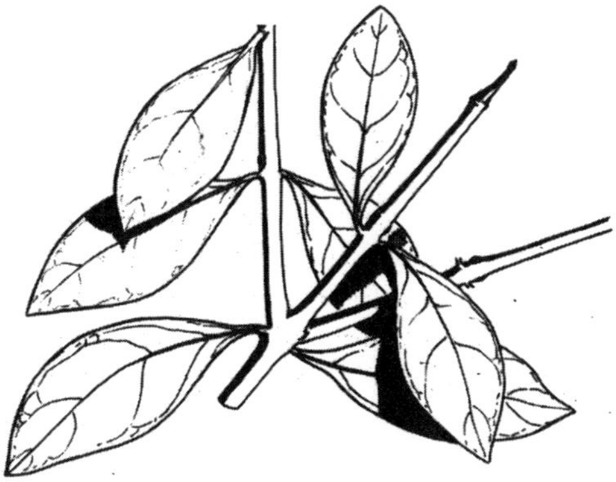

Fig. 8.3 Leaves of henna

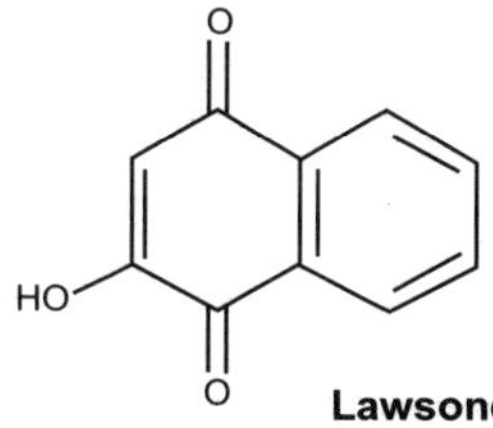

Lawsone

Henna is one of the oldest known cosmetics. Traditionally, it was used as a hair dye and in decorating finger nails, palms and soles, because of its cooling effect.

Chemical constituents

The fresh leaves contain glycosides that on hydrolysis yield a hydroxyl napthaquinone compound (2, 5-dihydroxy-1, 4 napthoquinone) called lawsone. This substance may be extracted from the leaf using sodium bicarbonate. The dried leaves contain about 1% lawsone. Lawsone is a natural orange dye that stains protein fibres. Henna also contains flavanoids, coumarins, xanthones, phenolic glycosides, fats, resins and tannins.

Uses

Henna is used as a colouring agent for hair, nails, soles of the feet and palms of hands. Thiol groups present in lawsone bind strongly with the keratin in hair and nail tissue. Henna is also used in the preparation of shampoos and hair lotions. Ayurveda recommends the use of henna in the treatment of skin ailments, burns and wounds. An essential oil obtained from the flowers of the henna plant is used in perfumery.

Henna leaves have an astringent action. A paste of the leaves is used to cool burning sensation in the feet and to treat headache. A decoction of henna leaves is also used for gargling to treat sore throat.

8.4 ALOE VERA

Biological source

It is obtained after eliminating the outermost tissue of the leaf of various species of aloe such as *Aloe berbadensis* and *Aloe vera* belonging to the Liliaceae family.

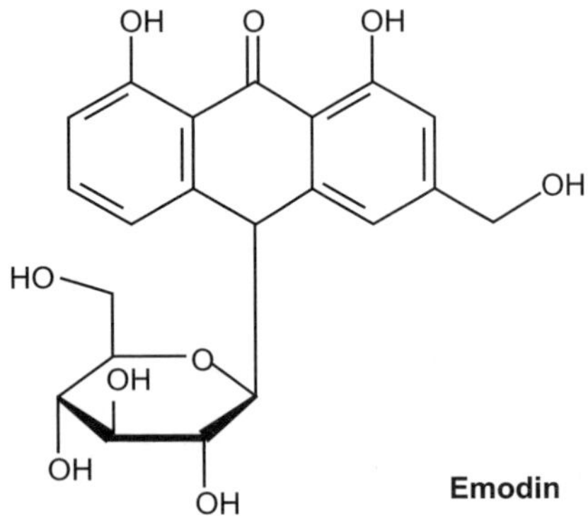

Emodin

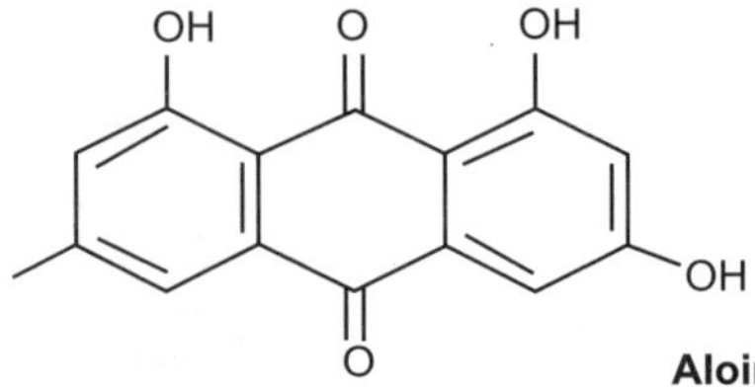

Aloin

Collection of the latex

Aloe is obtained from the mucilage of transversely cut leaves. This juice is present in the large pericyclic cells and occasionally in the adjacent parenchyma. Mucilage is present in the central region, which occupies three-fourths of the diameter of the leaf.

Due to its cellular composition, each and every cell has to be punctured to collect aloe. Subsequently, the mucilage from the leaf surface must be collected carefully. The collected product is filtered to remove the cellular impurities. Stainless steel strainers are usually employed, as the pH of the mucilage is acidic.

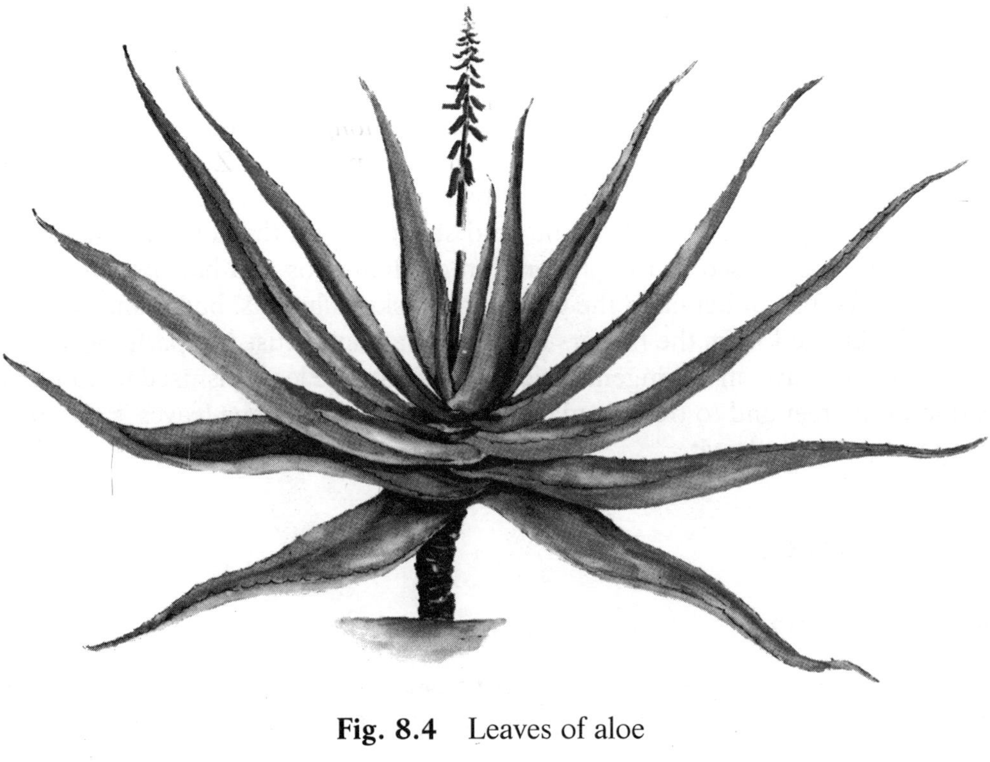

Fig. 8.4 Leaves of aloe

Chemical constituents

Aloe vera mucilage contains several amino acids, vitamins, minerals, enzymes and a polysaccharide containing glucomannan. Superoxide dismutase, glyoxylase I and glyoxylase II are the important enzymes present in aloe vera. The major fraction of the mucilage is called Acemannan. The most important anthraquinones, emodin and aloin have analgesic, anti-bacterial and anti-viral properties.

Uses

Aloe vera is a common ingredient of cosmetic preparations used for moisturizing the skin, such as, sun tan oils, lotions, soaps, shaving creams and gels. It is also useful in skin care products because of its anti-inflammatory, anti-bacterial and anti-fungal properties.

Aloe vera is used in the treatment of acne, insect bites, psoriasis, allergy and radiation burns in formulations such as creams, ointments and lotions. It is also used in treating gum sores caused by the use of dentures. It has also been used in the treatment of leukorrhoea.

8.5 TURMERIC

Biological source

It consists of fresh or dried rhizomes of *Curcuma longa* (*Curcuma domestica*) which contains not less than 4% volatile oils. Curcuma belongs to the Zingiberaceae family.

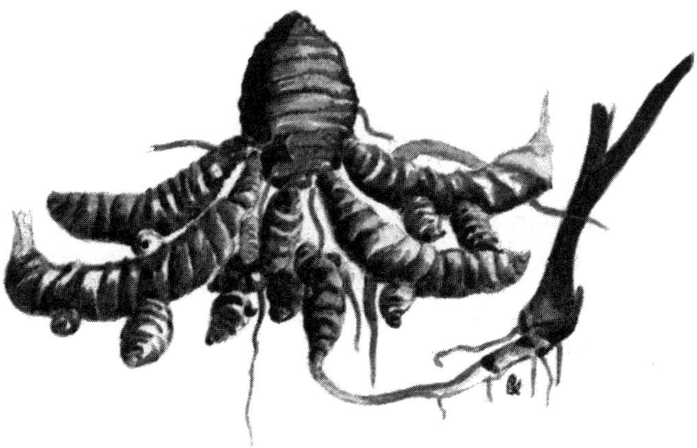

Fig 8.5 Rhizomes of turmeric

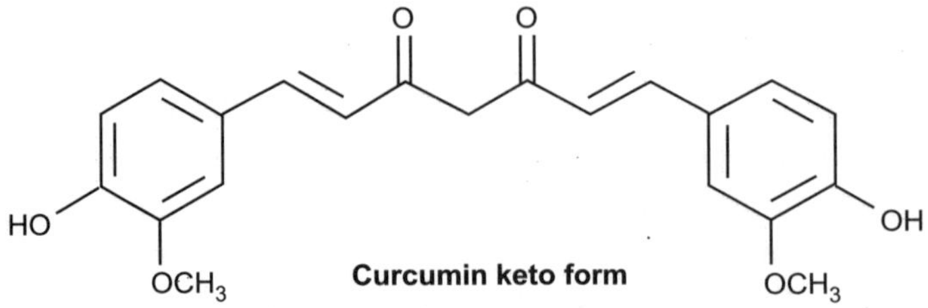

Curcumin keto form

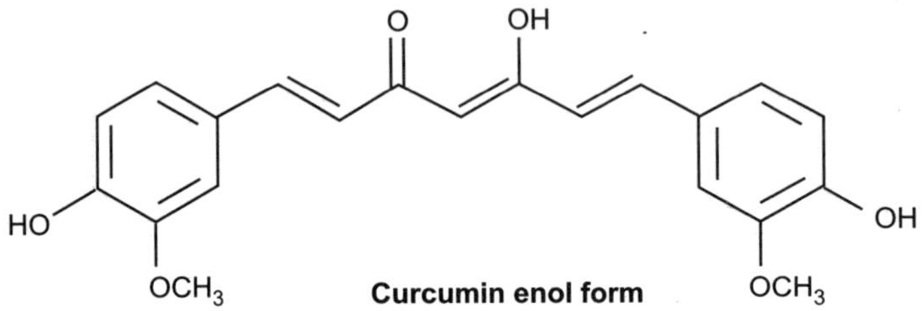

Curcumin enol form

Chemical constituents

Curcumin, a natural yellow pigment is the major constituent. It is a mixture of curcumin I, curcumin II and curcumin III. Curcumin dissolves in alcohol giving a deep yellow solution; on the addition of an alkali the colour changes to reddish brown. Turmeric also contains a volatile oil, resin, starch and sugars.

Turmeric has been found to contain mono and sesquiterpenes and derivatives obtained from their oxidation, such as, alcohol and ketones. The volatile oil mainly contains α- and β-phellandrene, camphor, zinziberene and β-curcumins.

Uses

Turmeric is widely used in cosmetics due to its broad spectrum anti-inflammatory and anti-microbial action. It has strong bleaching action on the skin. The bright yellow colour of turmeric makes it a good colouring agent. It also protects the skin due to its strong anti-oxidant action.

Turmeric has been traditionally used in the treatment of liver disorders and gall stones. Both curcumin I and II have shown significant cholagogue as well as choleretic actions. Turmeric is used in many Indian homes as the first line of treatment for coughs. Besides adding colour and flavour to cooking, turmeric also has appetite-stimulating properties.

8.6 SANDALWOOD OIL

Biological source

It is obtained by the distillation of the heart wood of *Santalum album* belonging to the Santalaceae family.

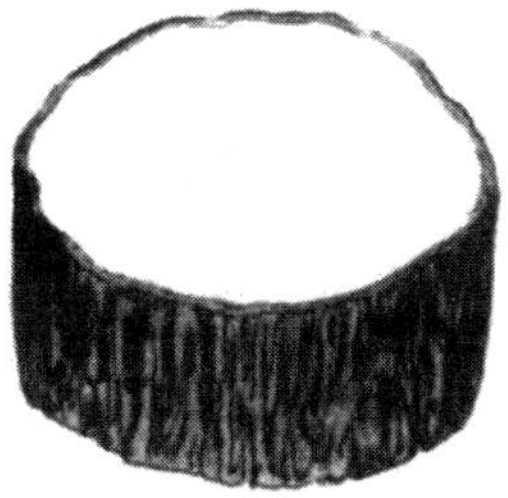

Fig. 8.6 Wood of sandalwood

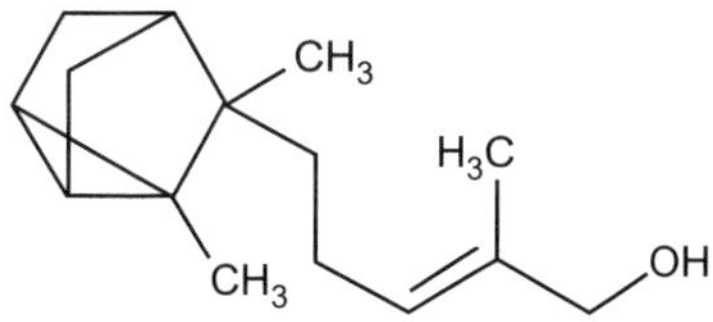

Santolol

Characteristics

The sweet, woody odour of sandalwood oil makes it a popular choice for use in perfumes, especially the expensive varieties. Besides exhibiting excellent blending properties, sandalwood oil is also a good fixative for other perfumes due to the presence of santalols.

Chemical constituents

It consists of two isomeric sesquiterpene alcohols, namely, α-santalol and β-santalol. It also contains an aldehyde, santalal, and other compounds such as santalone, santalene, santene and santenone.

Uses

Sandalwood oil has a delicate and characteristic aroma which makes it an ideal perfume. It is used to cool the body from the effects of sun stroke. The anti-inflammatory and soothing actions of sandalwood oil are useful in products used to treat acne. It also has strong astringent and germicidal effects because of which it is used as a skin protective.

When sandalwood oil is used for massaging or the vapours are inhaled through a vaporizer, it has a sedative action which is useful in the treatment of anxiety and depression. Its mild antiseptic and diuretic action render it useful in the treatment of urinary problems such as dysuria (painful micturition) and cystitis, and in reducing the frequency of micturition. Besides this, extracts of sandalwood are used in treating fever, headache and inflammations. It also has a stimulant and expectorant action. Sandalwood is used in the manufacture of incense sticks and traditional perfumes such as rose attars.

8.7 GLYCYRRHIZIN

Biological source

It is the triterpenoidal saponin obtained from *Glycyrrhiza glabra* of the Leguminosae family.

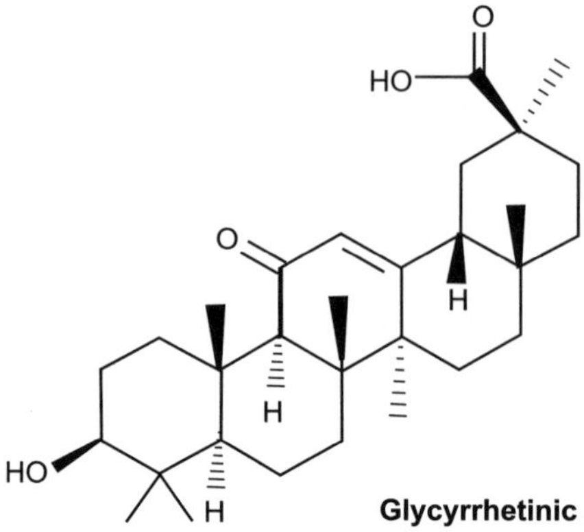

Glycyrrhetinic acid

Glycyrrhizin is the chief constituent of liquorice. This is chemically the potassium and calcium salts of glycyrrhizic or glycyrrhizinic acid. On hydrolysis, this yields 18β- glycyrrhetic acid or glycyrrhetinic acid. Glycyrrhiza also contains other components such as sugars like glucose and sucrose, glycyramarin resin, asparagine and flavonoids like isoliqueretin which show a remarkable anti-gastric effect.

USES

Due to its demulcent action, it is used widely in skin care products such as soothing lotions to relieve inflammation and mild pain. Glycyrrhizin is mainly used as a sweetening and flavouring agent in the preparation of dentifrices such as toothpastes and toothpowders.

It is used as an anti-spasmodic and in the treatment of peptic ulcer due to the presence of isoliqueretin. Glycyrrhizin has strong mineralo-corticoid activity and is used as an anti-inflammatory drug. It is often used as a substitute for corticosteroids in the treatment of rheumatoid arthritis. It also has expectorant action.

Exercises

Long answers

1. What are the various functions of cosmetics? Explain the advantages of herbal cosmetics and write a note on drugs used in skincare.
2. Discuss the action of haircare agents and describe any one herbal hair conditioner.

Short answers

3. What are the advantages and applications of herbal cosmetics?
4. Discuss the role of soapnut in shampoos.
5. List the uses of turmeric and henna.
6. List the cosmetic uses of sandalwood oil.
7. What are the various uses of aloe vera?

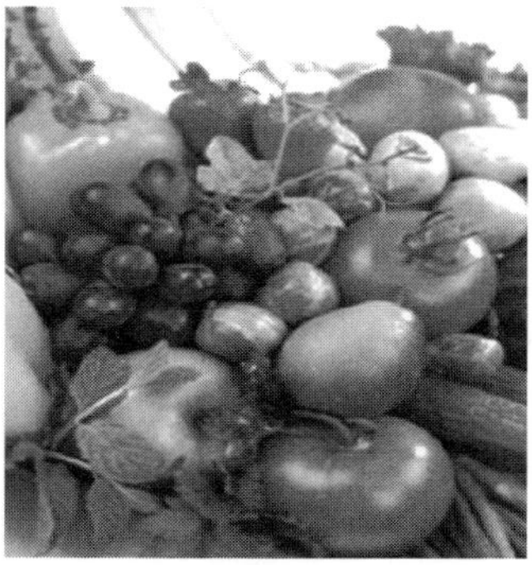

9

Enzymes

In This Chapter, You Will Learn

- The characteristics and mechanism of action of enzymes
- How enzymes are classified
- The factors affecting enzyme action
- The general methods used in the isolation of enzymes
- About some enzymes derived from plant and animal sources
- The methods of isolation and uses of some enzymes

Enzymes are defined as biological catalysts. They initiate and accelerate thousands of biochemical reactions in living cells. They are proteins and can be extracted from living tissues, purified and even crystallized.

Enzymes have an active site that helps bind substrate molecules; this binding catalyzes reactions because the molecules are held in the right spatial conformation to allow reactions to progress.

Purified enzymes can be used to carry out specific biochemical reactions outside the cells. Enzymes can also be variously modified through enzyme modelling and gene manipulations for a variety of purposes.

Enzyme engineering is a fast-growing application in the pharmaceutical market. Enzymes are the key to new processes because they are environment-friendly and reduce hazardous waste. Enzymatic reactions can occur under milder conditions, and at a faster rate, at the same time being highly specific. Therefore, the enzymatic process minimizes the time required for completion of a reaction.

General properties of enzymes

Enzymes have the following properties:

- They are the catalysts for many catabolic and anabolic reactions.

- They are proteinaceous and colloidal in nature.
- They are specific in their action on particular substrates and catalyze specific reactions.
- Their action is reversible; they can catalyze reactions in both directions.
- They get denatured by high temperature, pH, chemicals, x-rays and γ-rays.
- The rate of enzyme action is affected by temperature and pH.

Factors affecting enzyme action

Temperature

At 0°C enzyme action is low because the molecules move slowly. This results in a low collision frequency between the enzyme and substrate. As the temperature increases, the movement of molecules speeds up and hence, more 'enzyme–substrate complexes' are formed, leading to a greater degree of enzyme action. Maximum enzyme action is seen at 40°C. Beyond this temperature, enzyme action falls because the enzymes are rapidly denatured. When all the enzyme molecules are denatured, their action ceases.

pH

Enzyme action is optimum within a narrow range of pH, because a change in pH changes the hydrogen bonds involved in the tertiary shape of enzymes. As a result, the shape of the active site also changes and the substrate can no longer bind to the active site, thereby reducing enzyme action. A major pH change stops enzyme action by causing denaturation of the enzyme.

Human intracellular enzymes work best at 37°C and pH 7.

Concentration of substrate

The rate of an enzyme-catalyzed reaction depends on the concentration of both the enzyme and the substrate. As the concentration of either is increased, the rate of reaction increases. For a given enzyme concentration, the rate of reaction increases with increasing concentration of the substrate up to a point, above which any further increase in the substrate concentration produces no significant change in reaction rate. This is because the active sites of the enzyme are completely saturated with substrate. These enzyme–substrate complexes have to dissociate before the active sites are free to accommodate new substrate molecules.

Concentration of enzyme

The rate of reaction is proportional to the concentration of the enzyme, provided that the substrate concentration is high and the temperature and pH are kept constant.

Classification

Enzymes are classified by the International Union of Biochemistry into six classes based on the type of reaction catalyzed (Table 9.1).

Table 9.1 Classification of enzymes

Enzyme code	Group	Reaction catalyzed	Examples
1	Oxidoreductases	Oxidation–reduction	Dehydrogenases, oxidases
2	Transferases	Transfer of functional group	Transaminases
3	Hydrolases	Hydrolysis	Lipase, amylase, peptidase
4	Lyases	Non-hydrolytic addition or removal of groups	Decarboxylases
5	Isomerases	Intramolecular rearrangements (isomerization)	Mutase
6	Ligases	Synthesis of new bonds with simultaneous breakdown of ATP	Synthetases

USE OF ENZYMES IN THERAPY

Dr Edward Howell's work in the 1920s and 1930s serves as the foundation of enzyme therapy. Howell proposed that enzymes from foods help to pre-digest the food in the stomach. He advocated that large amounts of plant enzymes should be consumed to reduce the utilization of the body's digestive enzymes, which could then be directed towards other metabolic reactions.

Four categories of plant enzymes are considered useful for the process of pre-digestion: protease, amylase, lipase, and cellulase. Cellulase is particularly helpful because it is not produced within the human body.

Animal enzymes, such as pepsin, are more effective in the duodenum. They are often used for the treatment of non-digestive ailments.

Enzyme supplements can be extracted from plants such as pineapple and papaya and also from the organs of cows and pigs. Such supplements may be administered in either tablet or capsule form. Pancreatic enzymes may also be administered parenterally. The dosage varies according to the indication. For non-digestive ailments, the supplements should be consumed about an hour before a meal so that they can be quickly absorbed into the bloodstream. For digestive ailments, the supplements act best if taken immediately before meals, along with a large amount of liquid. A few important enzymes are discussed in the following sections.

9.1 PAPAIN

BIOLOGICAL SOURCE

It consists of the dried and purified latex of the fruit of *Carica papaya* belonging to the family of Caricaceae.

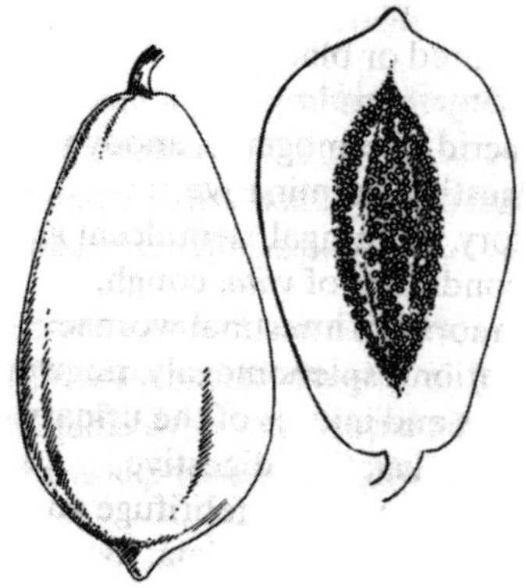

Fig. 9.1 Fruit of papaya

Description

It is a tree with a single, large stem that grows to a height of about 5–10 m. It has leaves that are spirally arranged and limited to the top of the trunk; the lower part of the trunk bears conspicuous scars where leaves and fruit were borne. The leaves are large, 50–70 cm in diameter, deeply palmately lobed with 7 lobes. The flowers of the papaya plant are smaller and sticky, appearing on the axils of the leaves. These flowers later mature into fruits that are large—about 15–45 cm long with a diameter of 10–30 cm. The ripening of the fruit can be detected from the softness of its skin and the change of colour from amber to orange.

Method of preparation

The latex is collected from fruits which are mature, but have a green skin. The best time for collection is during the morning on misty or cloudy days, or immediately after a spell of rain. The best season is during the period of both warm temperature and high humidity. Shallow incisions are made on four sides of the fully grown, unripe fruit. The latex is allowed to flow for a few seconds after which it immediately coagulates. This latex is collected into aluminium trays and immediately processed. Any delay will lead to loss of its enzymatic activity. Incisions are repeated at weekly intervals until the latex no longer exudes out. Extraneous matter can be cleared out by passing the latex through sieves. Potassium metabisulphite, an anti-oxidant, is added in the proportion 5 g to 1 kg of latex. Sun drying of the latex gives the lowest grade powder which appears cream-brown and has least activity; the product obtained from artificial drying is of a better grade. To prepare papain flakes, the latex is usually dried in batches of at least 500 kg (which will produce 50 kg of flakes). The latex is filtered and centrifuged to produce a 45% solid concentration. This latex is taken in a tank and whisked to produce a homogeneous liquid. This liquid is filtered through muslin cloth to remove waxy components and poured into shallow trays. The trays are placed in a drying house and dried at 60°C for 3 to 4 days or until the flakes dry completely. Oven drying after filtration gives a powder or flakes with lighter colour and greater activity levels than that produced by sun drying. Advanced methods of drying, such as spray drying, may also be used.

Purification

The flakes are purified by general purification and separation technique of precipitation and solution. Crude papain is dissolved in water and then precipitated using alcohol. It can also be purified by affinity chromatography.

Description

Papain is a light brown or white amorphous powder with typical odour and taste.

Chemical nature

Papain contains several proteolytic enzymes. It is soluble in water and glycerine. It is also known as 'vegetable pepsin' because it contains enzymes similar to pepsin. However, unlike pepsin, it can act in acid, neutral or alkaline media. It shows maximum activity at a pH of 5–6. Some of the enzymes found in papain are:

- Peptidase I which converts proteins to dipeptides and polypeptides
- Renin-like coagulation enzyme which acts on casein present in milk
- Amylolytic enzymes
- Clotting enzymes similar to pectase
- An enzyme with mild activity on fats

The strength of papain depends on the method of manufacture. Generally, papain can digest about 35 times its own weight of lean meat. It is therefore widely used as a meat tenderizer. The best grade of papain can digest about 300 times its own weight of egg albumin.

Identification

It turns an aqueous solution of potassium permanganate colourless and causes curdling of milk.

Uses

It digests proteins because of its pepsin-like action. Hence, it is included in various digestive preparations. It is also used in such preparations in combination with other enzymes like amylases.

- It acts as an anti-inflammatory agent and helps in healing wounds.
- It is used along with antibiotics to treat skin diseases.
- It is used to heal the cut made during episiotomy (surgical incision of the vulva for obstetric purposes).
- It is an important ingredient of solutions used in cleaning soft contact lenses.
- It also has industrial applications. It is used in tenderizing meat, clarifying beverages, making cheese, softening textiles and tanning leather.

Chymopapain

It is also found in the latex from papaya and is chemically related to papain. It is a protein, comprising 218 amino acids. It is used in the treatment of sciatica due to herniated lumbar disc. When no other treatment is possible, it is injected into the intervertebral disc. However, this administration should be done only by highly trained personnel due to the associated risk of anaphylactic shock.

9.2 BROMELAIN

Biological source

It consists of a mixture of proteolytic enzymes obtained from the stem and ripened fruits of the pineapple plant, *Ananas comosus*, belonging to the Bromeliaceae family.

Pineapple is a perennial plant that grows to a height of about 1.0–1.5 m and has 30 or more trough-shaped, pointed leaves, 30–100 cm long, arranged around a thick stem. The pineapple is an example of a multiple fruit where each of the helically-arranged flowers along the axis produces a fleshy fruit. This in turn gets pressed against the fruits of adjacent flowers, giving rise to the appearance of a single fleshy fruit.

Description

It is odourless but sometimes slightly putrid smelling, buff powder that has an irritating taste. It is slightly soluble in water and insoluble in organic solvents such as ether, chloroform and alcohol. It is a protein-digesting and milk-clotting enzyme.

Method of preparation

It is mainly produced in Thailand, Taiwan, and other tropical countries where pineapple is grown widely.

The fruit is harvested and the stem is peeled, crushed and pressed. The juice so extracted contains the bromelain enzyme which is subjected to further processing to purify and concentrate the enzyme.

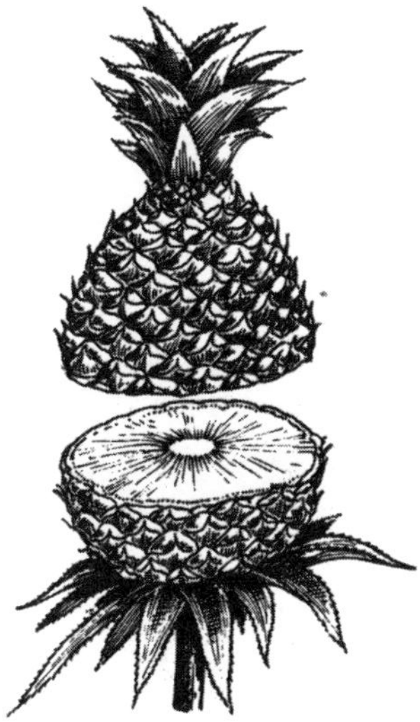

Fig. 9.2 Fruit of pineapple

USES

Bromelain is a useful anti-inflammatory agent for soft tissues and in cases of oedema caused by surgery or injury. It is believed to act by blocking some pro-inflammatory metabolites which speed up the inflammatory process. It also reduces the migration of neutrophils to sites of acute inflammation.

- It has been investigated for treatment of traveller's diarrhoea.
- It is used in the commercial production of protein hydrolyzates and as a meat tenderizer.
- It is used in the leather industry.
- Bromelain is being investigated for its use in the treatment of conditions such as bruising, gout, arthritis, haemorrhoids, menstrual pain and autoimmune disorders as well as AIDS.

9.3 STREPTOKINASE

It is the purified bacterial protein elaborated by group C β-hemolytic streptococci (*Streptococcus pyogenes*). *S. pyogenes* is a spherical Gram-positive bacterium growing in long chains. When cultured on blood agar plates it produces large zones of complete disruption of erythrocytes and causes release of hemoglobin. Hence, it is also known as Group A β-hemolytic streptococcus.

Activity

Although streptokinase does not have direct enzymatic action on plasminogen, it binds to plasminogen in a 1:1 ratio, causing a molecular conformational change to activate the complex. This cleaves the bonds on other plasminogen molecules and converts them to plasmin, the fibrinolytic enzyme. Plasmin degrades both fibrinogen and fibrin clots and other plasma proteins. This enzyme causes activation of a fibrinolytic enzyme in human serum that breaks fibrin into smaller fragments. Thus, the blood clots and fibrinous exudates dissolve quickly.

Description

It is a sterile friable solid white powder, soluble in water with maximum activity at pH 7. Highly concentrated solutions are stable for about 6 hours at 4°C; dilute solutions are unstable.

Method of preparation

The fermentation process to produce streptokinase consists of the following steps:

1. Preparation of the medium
2. Fermentation
3. Purification
4. Purification by DEAE cellulose

Preparation of medium

Any of the following ingredients can be a suitable medium:

- Casein digest solution is prepared by dissolving casein in water and heating to 100°C and maintaining at the same temperature, until the solution is clear. The resulting solution is rapidly cooled to 15°C and filtered through a coarse filter paper. Toluene is added in small quantities for the purpose of preservation. It is stored for four days at 20°C and subsequently filtered to remove the insoluble material.
- Potassium dihydrogen phosphate
- Cysteine in 10% HCl
- Glycine
- Tryptophan
- Dextrose
- Uracil
- Vitamins such as nicotinic acid, pyridoxine, calcium pantothenate, thiamine hydrochloride and riboflavin

- Adenine sulphate
- Thioglycollic acid
- Potassium bicarbonate
- Trace elements such as magnesium sulphate, copper sulphate, manganese sulphate and ferrous sulphate

Fermentation

The sterilized medium is inoculated with seed inoculation of the bacterium *S. hemolyticus* which has a bacterial count of 20 billion/ml. Fermentation is carried out in a tank for 14 hours at 37°C. During this period, no pH adjustment, aeration or modifications should be made. Later, 50% dextrose solution is added and pH is adjusted to 6 at 15-minute intervals by using 5N NaOH. After each adjustment of pH, 50% dextrose solution is added. Fermentation is continued until the bacterial count stops increasing. This may take around 8 hours. At this stage, the fermentation medium would contain approximately 1000 units/ml.

Purification

The crude streptokinase is first dialyzed against phosphate buffer. It is then applied on modified cellulosic columns and eluted using phosphate buffer solutions of increasing pH and molarity (increasing pH from 5.8 to 8.5 and molarity from 0.005M to 0.1M) as both are very important factors in purification. At 0.1M concentration, streptokinase is eluted whereas a higher molarity leads to improper adsorption and separation. At pH greater than 8.5, the adsorption capacity of cellulose reduces drastically and at pH lesser than 5.8, streptokinase is completely precipitated. Impurities are eluted at pH 8 and at a molarity of 0.75.

Purification by DEAE cellulose

Crude streptokinase, phosphate buffer (0.2M) and DEAE cellulose, in the proportion of 3:2:1, are stirred for one hour and filtered. The cake that is obtained is washed using 0.025M phosphate buffer and stirred for 30 minutes. It is again filtered and the cake is suspended in 0.1M phosphate buffer with stirring for one hour. The filtrate collected will contain pure streptokinase.

USES

Streptokinase is used in the treatment of pulmonary embolism, deep vein thrombosis, arterial thrombosis and embolism, occlusion of arterio-venous cannula and coronary artery thrombosis.

The treatment with streptokinase is found to be most beneficial when it is administered early during the course of a myocardial infarction or other clotting episodes.

Side effects

The use of streptokinase has the following side effects.

- It leads to both peripheral and intracranial bleeding.
- It may also cause anaphylaxis and other allergic reactions.

Plasminogen–streptokinase complex can also be formed in vitro and chemically modified (anisolylated) to retain the stability of its enzymatic properties. Anisolylated plasminogen–streptokinase activated complex (APSAC) known as 'anistreptase' is used in the same manner as streptokinase.

Streptodornase

This is a related enzyme which acts directly on substrates such as deoxyribonucleoproteins and DNA, which are the main constituents of nuclei, and are also found in purulent exudates. Streptodornase splits these compounds into free purine bases and pyrimidine nucleosides, thereby decreasing the viscosity of the purulent exudates.

9.4 UROKINASE

Urokinase is an enzyme isolated from human urine, obtained from human kidney cells by tissue culture techniques or by recombinant DNA technology. There are two forms of this enzyme that have similar clinical effects but vary in their molecular weight.

Activity

It is a plasminogen activator that causes conversion of plasminogen to plasmin. Since plasmin has proteolytic action, it causes a breakdown of fibrin.

Method of preparation

It is obtained from human urine. The chemicals required include sodium benzoate, hydrochloric acid, benzoic acid and celite-505.

Human urine is mixed with 6% w/v sodium benzoate solution and dilute HCl is added to adjust the pH to 4.5. The heavy precipitate formed is stirred for about 20 minutes and kept for a further 30 minutes. The precipitate obtained is filtered through a Buchner funnel containing a filter paper pre-coated with benzoic acid crystals. Urokinase is adsorbed on the benzoic acid cake, which is later washed with saturated benzoic acid through a Buchner funnel to obtain a dry cake. The dry cake is then treated with a volume of acetone that is around 1.5 times the weight of the cake to dissolve the benzoic acid. This precipitates the enzyme by flocculation. The process can be speeded up by adding a small quantity of sodium benzoate.

The suspension obtained in the above step is filtered through a Buchner funnel fitted with a filter paper pre-coated with celite-505. The precipitate which gets adsorbed on the celite, is washed first with acetone and then with ether. The washed precipitate is air dried and urokinase is adsorbed on the celite.

The air-dried precipitate is suspended in 0.1M phosphate saline buffer of pH 6 and stirred to dissolve the urokinase. This is centrifuged and the extract is collected. The extract is passed through Amberlite XE-64 ion exchanger resin and the column is washed with phosphate saline buffer. The adsorbate is eluted with 0.5 M NaCl.

The eluate obtained from chromatography is subjected to dialysis through a viscose regenerated cellulose membrane against distilled water. The product obtained from dialysis is then lyophilized to obtain urokinase.

Uses

Urokinase has the following applications:

- It is useful in treating acute massive pulmonary embolism, rheumatic heart disease, myocardial infarction and coronary artery thrombosis.
- It is useful in the treatment of venous thrombosis.
- It is also used to dissolve fibrin and blood clots present in the anterior chamber of the eye.
- It also has a role in the treatment of frostbite and acute gangrene.

Urokinase is less antigenic than other enzymes, possibly due to its origin from a human source. Hence, there is a reduced probability of serious allergic reactions.

9.5 HYALURONIDASE

This enzyme enhances the diffusion and absorption of injected fluids.

Biological source

It is present in certain tissues, particularly in the testicular and spleen tissue. It is also present in some types of pneumococci and certain hemolytic streptococci.

Activity

This enzyme hydrolyzes hyaluronic acid, a type of lipo-polysaccharide found in intercellular ground substance. By hydrolyzing the glucose amidic bonds it causes a temporary reduction in the viscosity of the cellular cement. This promotes diffusion of the injected fluids of localized transudates or exudates and hence, the absorption increases. It is also known as a spreading factor or spreading agent because it causes a greater spreading of materials in tissue spaces.

METHOD OF PREPARATION

Hyaluronidase is produced by a process that involves fermentation of the source organism, *Streptococcus hyalurolytics*. This organism is cultivated for 48–96 hours at a temperature of 27–30°C under aeration.

Preparation of culture medium

The following ingredients are dissolved in 100 ml of water, sterilized at 120°C for 15 minutes and the pH adjusted to 7.2.

Glucose 25%
Carmine 1%
Ammonium sulphate 0.5%
Yeast extract 0.25%
Potassium hydrogen phosphate 0.1%

Inoculation and fermentation

The sterilized medium is inoculated with *S. hyalurolytics*. This organism is pre-cultured in the same medium for 48 hours at 30°C with constant shaking.

Isolation of product

Cells are removed by filtration. Enzyme activity is measured in turbidity reduction units (TRU). The activity of the enzyme in the culture filtrate is 13 TRU/ml. For the isolation of the product, the pH is adjusted to 5 and subsequently fractionated between 40%–60% saturation with ammonium sulphate. The precipitate is collected and dissolved in suitable amount of water.

Purification of the product

It is done by gel filtration (molecular sieving).

USES

- Hyaluronidase is used to enhance the dispersion and absorption of injected drugs.
- It is used in improving the re-absorption of radio-opaque drugs.
- It has been found to decrease post-operative oedema and ecchymosis.
- It is used to increase penetration of drugs like penicillin into the mucous membrane.

Hyaluronidase should not be injected into infected or cancerous areas because it may lead to spreading of the offending material.

9.6 ASPARAGINASE

These are a group of enzymes which possess anti-tumour activity. Their natural sources are diverse, ranging from bacteria such as *E. coli* and Mycobacteria, fungi such as penicillin and yeast and higher plants such as the rootlets of barley to animal sources such as the serum of guinea pig.

Depending on their source, the various asparaginases differ in their molecular weights and substrate specificity.

Activity

Asparaginase causes the deamination of asparagine to aspartic acid and ammonia. This reaction enables the anti-neoplastic activity of asparaginase in two ways:

- Some tumour cells require asparagine (a non-essential amino acid) for their growth. When asparaginase causes deamination of this amino acid and depletes its level, it leads to cell death and a subsequent regression of the tumour.
- Aspartic acid and ammonia produced during deamination also have an inhibitory effect on tumour cells.

However, asparaginases can act only on specific tumours. Hence, in vitro tests with tumours are required prior to their usage. Some important tests are the degree of L-asparagin synthetase activity in the tumour, the effect of L-asparagine on the growth of the tumour in tissue culture and the effects of asparaginases on the viability of tumour cells in tissue culture. The results of these tests determine their effectiveness in treatment.

Method of preparation

Isolation

The enzyme is isolated from guinea pig serum and purified. The serum of the guinea pig is collected by centrifugation. Only 5 ml can be collected from each animal and hence, a number of animals have to be used. These samples are pooled together and the enzyme is precipitated using sodium sulphate half saturation method (15 g/100 ml). This precipitate is then dissolved in ammonia-free distilled water and subjected to column chromatography by passing it through a column of calcium phosphate gel to remove impurities. The effluent portion is stored at 10°C and then dialyzed against multiple changes of 0.0005M phosphate buffer of pH 7 at 0°C for 48 hours. DEAE cellulose column chromatography and elution with 0.0005M phosphate buffer at pH 7 gives the pure product. The efficient peak containing asparaginase is collected. Further purification is achieved through electrophoresis. The final product is concentrated and stored at –10°C.

Preparation from E. coli

As *E. coli* is also a major source for asparaginase, *E. coli* BATcc 11303 is transferred from stock culture to fresh nutrient medium layer and allowed to grow for 18 hours at 37°C. Then, the surface growth is transferred to the culture medium containing the following:

Peptone 2%
Dextrose 1%
Yeast extract 0.6%
Potassium dihydrogen phosphate

Amino acids such as leucine, glycine, alanine and methionine are useful in improving the yield and the pH is adjusted to 7.5.

Fermentation

The sterile medium is inoculated with organisms and incubated at 37°C for 18 hours with moderate aeration without dissolved oxygen. The degree of aeration should be carefully controlled as excessive aeration causes reduced yield. It is again cultured by transferring the organisms to a larger quantity and cultivated for 18 to 24 hours.

Extraction

The cells are separated and freeze dried, then homogenized with 20 ml of 0.05M TRES buffer of pH 8. This is centrifuged; the supernatant is collected and extracted with 0.5M manganese chloride. The precipitate is discarded and the liquid is precipitated using ammonium sulphate to obtain the final asparaginase.

Purification

The precipitate of asparaginase is dissolved in purified water and then subjected to dialysis against distilled water. The solution is concentrated at –5°C. Methanol is added and the precipitate obtained after centrifugation is collected.

Asparaginase can also be produced by the use of recombinant DNA technology.

USES

- Asparaginase is used in the treatment of acute lymphoblastic leukemia.
- It has also been found useful in the treatment of certain mast cell tumors.
- It is used in management of non-Hodgkin's lymphoma.

SUMMARY

- Enzymes are biological catalysts for various reactions, both in vitro and in vivo.
- Various factors like concentration of substrate and enzyme, temperature and pH affect the activity of enzymes.
- Due to their digestive abilities, enzymes such as papain, bromelain, streptokinase, hyaluronidase and urokinase are used in the treatment of various disorders.

Exercises

Long answers

1. Discuss the chemical nature and uses of papain.
2. Discuss the chemical nature and uses of bromelain.
3. Describe the method of preparation of urokinase and streptokinase.

Short answers

4. Briefly describe the method of production of papain.
5. Describe the method of isolation of bromelain.
6. What are the uses of streptokinase?

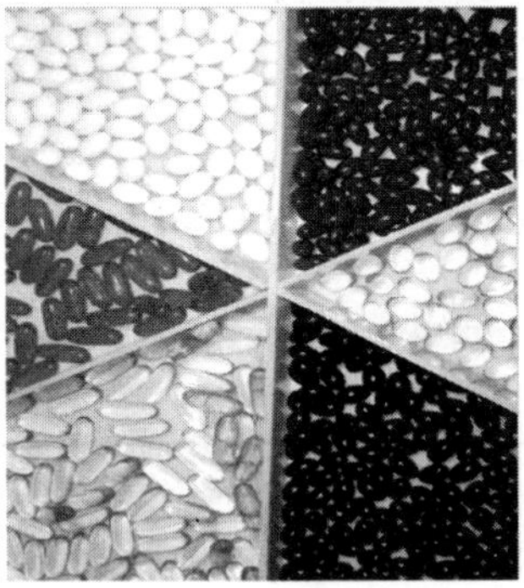

10 Nutraceuticals

In This Chapter, You Will Learn

- Various types of nutraceuticals and their characteristics
- Sources and potential benefits of various classes of nutraceuticals
- The biological source, chemical constituents and uses of a few nutraceuticals

Stephen de Felice, Founder–Chairman, Foundation for Innovation in Medicine (FIM), coined the term 'nutraceuticals' in 1989. It refers to foods that have some medical benefits, such as, prevention and treatment of diseases. Such foods are also known as functional foods. Commercially marketed nutraceuticals consist of both traditional and non-traditional foods.

Definition

A 'nutraceutical' is defined as a substance which has, in addition to its nutritional value as food, the capacity to provide health benefits by preventing disease or promoting well being.

Nutraceuticals are mainly associated with the prevention or treatment of heart disease, cancer, hypertension, diabetes, osteoporosis, arthritis and neural tube defects. The food products used as nutraceuticals include antioxidants, prebiotics, probiotics, omega-3 fatty acids and certain dietary fibres. Except probiotics, all these components are present in fruits, vegetables and different types of herbal foods. Table 10.1 lists some common classes of nutraceuticals, their source and health benefits.

10.1 IMPORTANT CLASSES OF NUTRACEUTICALS

ANTIOXIDANTS

They contain vitamins E, C, A, and β-carotenes. They are present in some fruits, vegetables, fixed oils and fish. The antioxidants present in them act by one of two mechanisms. They either prevent the synthesis of oxygen-free radicals or have a scavenging effect to trap these radicals. Garlic for example, contains a compound *S*-allylcysteine sulphoxide (SACS) which acts by scavenging the free radicals. Lipid membranes are rich in vitamin E, which is an important radical trapper. It therefore proves useful in the clinical treatment of cardiac damage and neoplasms. Selenium is another important anti-carcinogenic material that prevents lipid peroxidation induced by oxygen radicals. Ascorbic acid is yet another strong antioxidant; it acts as a scavenger of superoxide radicals.

POLYUNSATURATED FATTY ACIDS (PUFA)

These are a common component of many vegetable oils, such as, safflower oil, mustard oil and soybean oil, and marine almonds. The vegetable oils are rich in PUFA belonging to the linoleic group (omega-6-type), whereas marine fish contain PUFA belonging to the linolenic groups (omega-3-type). Omega-3 fatty acids have a significant role in preventing atherosclerosis due to their ability to increase HDL levels and reduce levels of LDL and VLDL. They also help reduce the formation of thromboxane and cause increased fibrinolysis. This improves the flowability of the blood. Besides, the thromboxane lowering action leads to a strong anti-inflammatory capacity, due to which it is used in the treatment of arthritis.

PROBIOTICS

These are living microorganisms that have a capacity to improve the intestinal–microbial balance. They can be taken with or without food and help in better functioning of the large intestine. Probiotics include lactobacilli species such as *L. acidophillus* and Bifidobacterium species. The action of these organisms is attributed to their ability to synthesize certain compounds which can inhibit the growth of harmful bacteria in the large intestine. Examples of probiotics include products like sour milk and yoghurt.

PREBIOTICS

These compounds protect the probiotics from attack by the digestive enzymes and acids in the upper part of the gastro-intestinal tract. They can also promote the growth of selective colonic probiotic bacteria. The best known prebiotic is *inulin*, a polyfructose compound obtained mainly from the roots of *Cichorium intibus* (chicory). Chicory, a

Table 10.1 Classification and uses of nutraceuticals

Class/Components	Source	Probable benefits	Structure
Carotenoids			
Beta carotene	Carrots and fruits	Neutralize free radicals which can damage cells; reinforce the cellular antioxidant defence mechanism	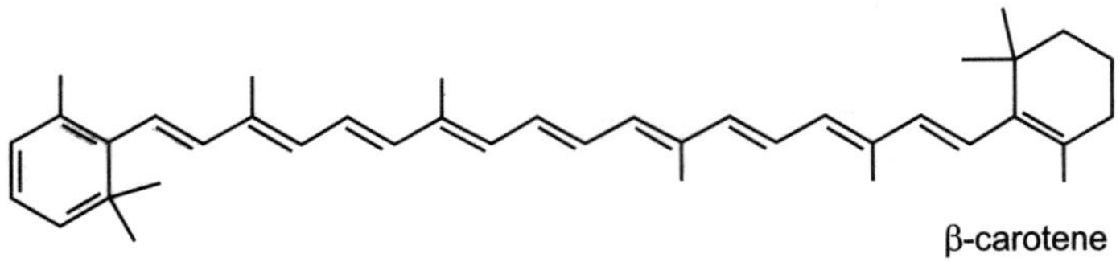 β-carotene
Lycopene	Tomatoes and processed tomato products	Contribute to the maintenance of a healthy prostate	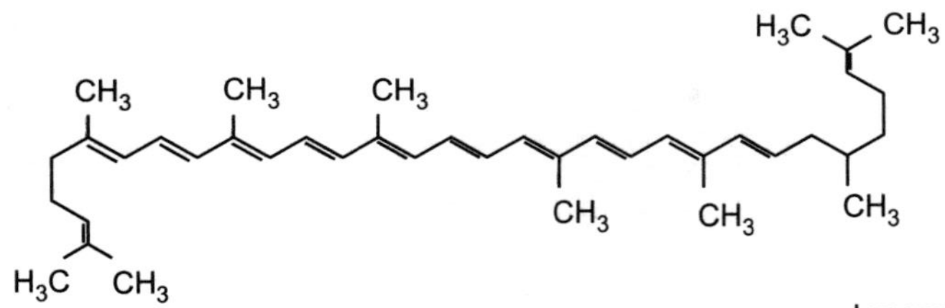 Lycopene
Fatty acids			
Monounsaturated fatty acids	Macadamia nuts, hazelnuts, cashewnuts, almonds and hickorynuts	Decrease the risk of coronary heart disease	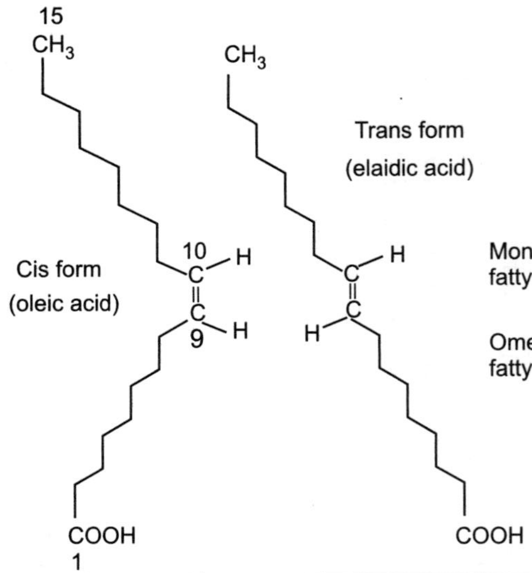 Mono-unsaturated fatty acids
Omega-3 fatty acids	Fish oil, walnut, flax seed, sunflower seed.	Reduce pain and discomfort due to artitis Protect against heart disease	Omega-3 and Omega-6 fatty acids

Class/Components	Source	Probable benefits	Structure
Polyphenolics			
Flavonols	Onions, apples, tea and broccoli	Neutralize free radicals which can damage cells, augment cellular antioxidant defence	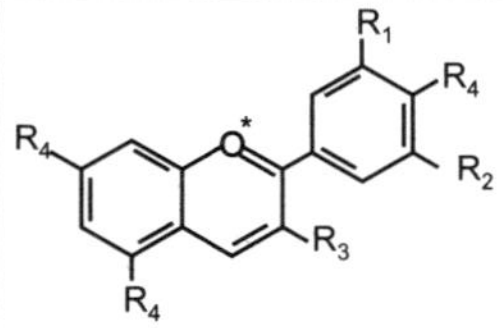 **Anthocyanins / Anthocyanidins** 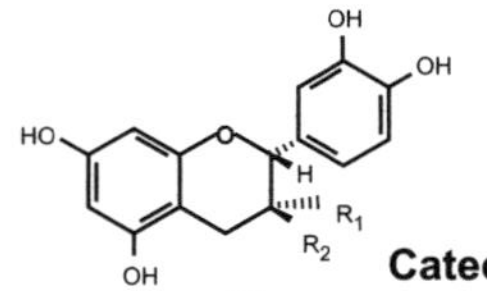 **Catechins**
Anthocyanins	Berries, green tea, potato and cherries	Antioxidant, anti-cancer anti-inflammatory, anti-diabetic	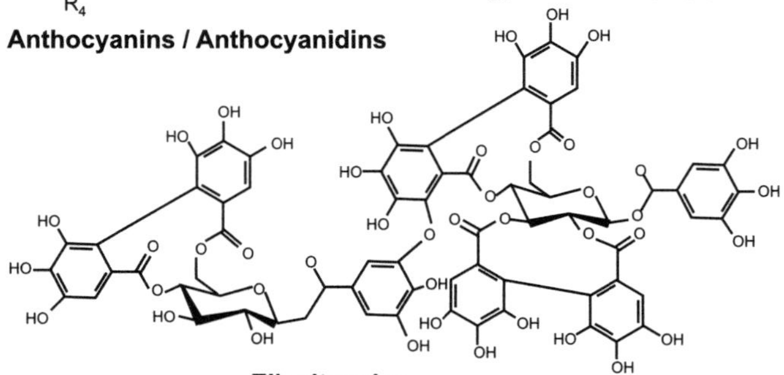 **Ellagitannins** 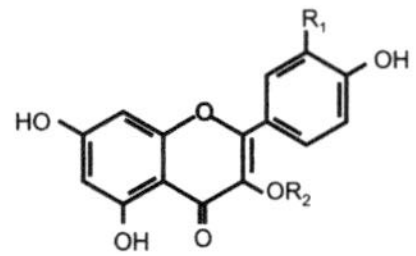 **Flavonols** 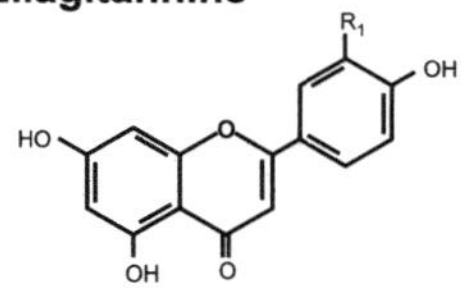 **Flavones** 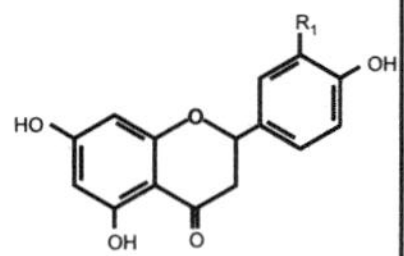 **Flavonones**
Dietary fibre			
Insoluble fibre	Wheat bran	Contribute to the maintenance of digestive health	
Isothiocyanates			
Sulphoraphane	Cauliflower, cabbage, broccoli and horse radish	Enhance detoxification of undersirable cells, augment cellular antioxidant defence	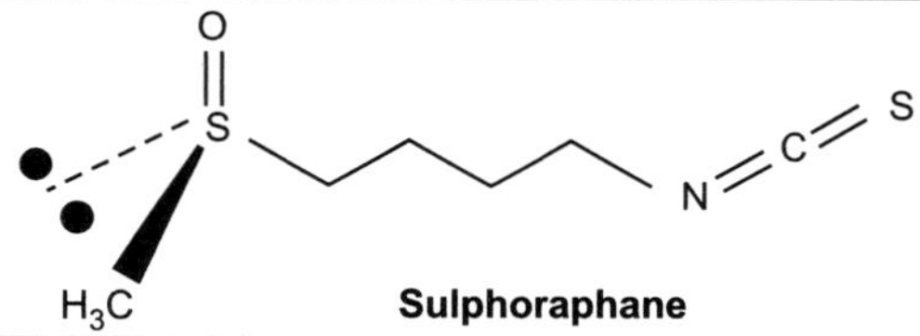 **Sulphoraphane**

Table 10.1 Continued

Class/Components	Source	Probable benefits	Structure
Plant stanols/sterols Stanol/sterol esters	Fortified table spreads, stanol ester dietary supplements	Decrease risk of coronary heart disease	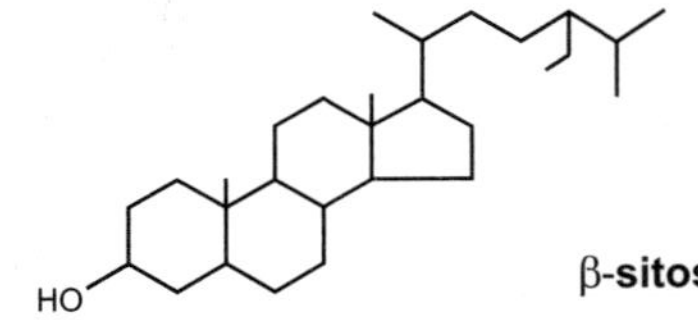 **β-sitostanol**
Phenols Caffeic acid and ferulic acid	Apples, pears, citrus fruits and some vegetables	Bolster cellular antioxidant defense, contribute to maintenance of healthy heart	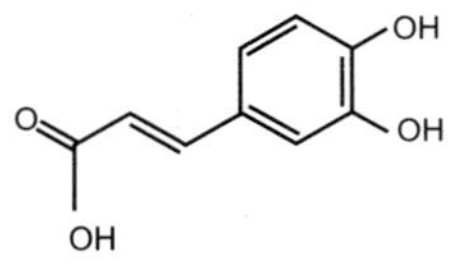 **Caffeic acid** 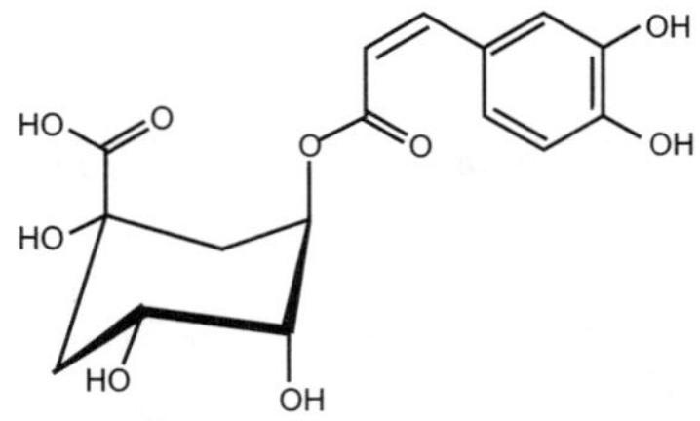 **Chlorogenic acid** 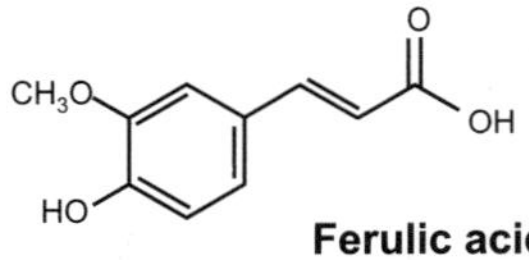 **Ferulic acid**
Polyols Sugar alcohols (xylitol, sorbitol, mannitol, lactitol)	Some chewing gums and other food applications	May reduce dental caries (cavities)	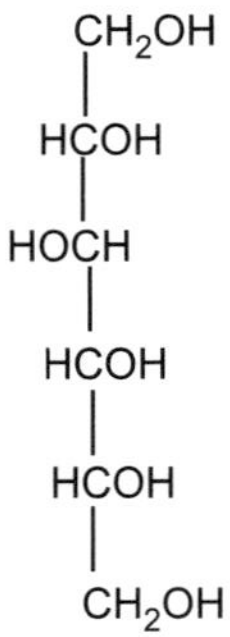 **Sorbitol** 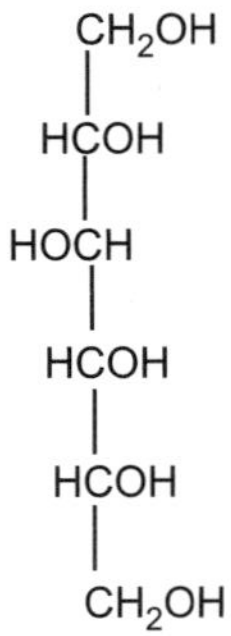 **D-Mannitol** 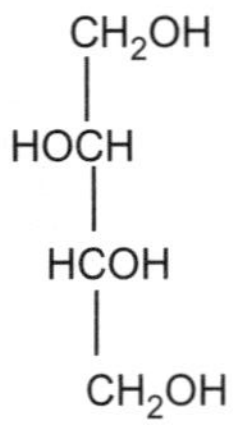 **Erythritol**

Class/Components	Source	Probable benefits	Structure
Prebiotics/probiotics Lactobacilli, bifidobacteria	Yogurt, other dairy and non-dairy applications	Improve gastrointestinal health and systematic immunity	
Soy protein	Soybeans and soy based foods	Decrease risk of coronary heart disease	
Phytoestrogens Isoflavones (diadzein, genistein)	Soybeans, and soy-based foods-flaxseed, garlic, dried apricots and dates, sesame seeds, multi grained bread and alfalfa sprout.	Contribute to healthy bones, brain and immune functions, maintain menopausal health in women	Isoflavones 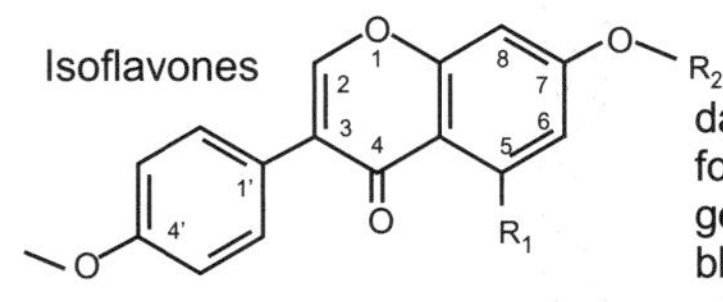 R R$_2$ daidzein H H formononetin H CH_3 genistein OH H blochanin A OH CH_3
Glucophenolates or thioglucosides	Brussel sprouts and watercress	Anti-cancer property, liver detoxification, effective in cardiovascular disease and arthritis, and improve immunity.	

Table 10.1 Continued

Class/ Components	Source	Probable benefits	Structure
Sulphides/thiols Dithiolthiones	Cruciferous vegetables: cabbage, broccoli and cauliflower Ginseng and satavari	Contribute to a healthy immune system	
Saponins	Ginseng and satavari	Anti-stress action, general tonic and adaptogen, galactogogue	
Thiosulphinates or cysteine sulphoxide	Garlic and onions	Anti-microbial action, reduce high blood pressure, inhibit platelet aggregation	

soluble dietary fibre is delivered intact to the colon because it is resistant to digestive enzymes. It undergoes fermentation due to the action of bacteria residing in the colon. The lactobacilli and bifidobacteria digest inulin and feed on it.

Dietary fibres

There are many non-digestible polysaccharides found in plant cell walls. These are referred to as dietary fibres, and can be of two types: soluble and insoluble. Soluble fibres are partially soluble in water and dissolve to form a gel, whereas the insoluble fibres are insoluble in water and therefore, pass through the digestive tract without any degradation. Both types of fibres form an important component of the diet and serve in maintaining the regularity of bowel movements. Yet another advantage of soluble fibres is that they play a role in lowering blood cholesterol levels, and therefore reduce the risk of heart attack. Oat meal, oat bran, nuts, cheese, legumes, apples and strawberries are rich in soluble fibres. Insoluble dietary fibres are present in whole wheat, carrots, cucumber, barley, tomatoes and brown rice.

10.2 GARLIC

Biological source

It is the fresh or dried bulb of *Allium sativum* belonging to the family Liliaceae.

Since ancient times, garlic has been used in cooking and traditional medicine. It has a typical spicy and pungent flavour that adds taste to food. The garlic bulb is made up of many fleshy parts called cloves. Oil can be obtained by steam distillation of the crushed fresh bulbs of garlic.

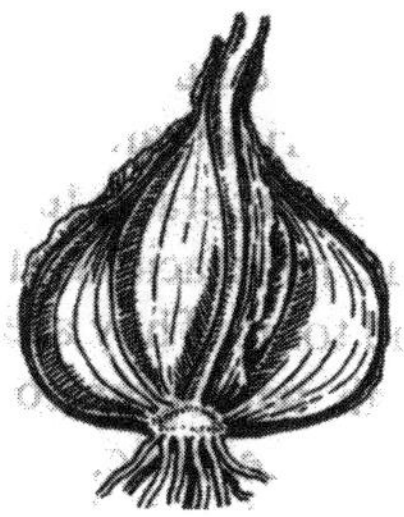

Fig. 10.1 Bulb of garlic

Chemical constituents

The pharmacological activity of garlic is due to the volatile oil content which is present in a proportion of about 0.1%–0.36%. Garlic is made up of numerous sulphur-containing compounds like alliin, allicin, ajoene, allylpropl, diallyl, trisulfide, sallylcysteine, vinyldithiines, *S*-allylmercaptocystein and others. In fact, it has the highest sulphur content when compared to other Allium species and that is responsible for most of its medicinal properties. Garlic also contains amino acids, selenium, glycosides and enzymes such as allinase, peroxidases and myrosinase among others. The typical odour of garlic is due to the action of the enzyme, allinase, on the sulphur-containing compound alliin. This enzyme is destroyed by heat, and hence, cooked garlic is not as effective as eating it raw, nor does it have as penetrating an odour. When garlic is cut or crushed, it releases the compound allicin by the action of allinase on alliin. Allicin shows maximum physiological activity.

Uses

- It has strong antibiotic action against a wide range of microorganisms and is commonly used in the treatment of cough and cold.
- It has been found useful in reducing blood pressure and helps to lower cholesterol levels, thus reducing the risk of cardiovascular diseases.
- Raw garlic has been used to treat skin ailments such as acne vulgaris.
- It has strong antioxidant action and is a natural mosquito repellent.
- Owing to its anti-carcinogenic properties, it has been found to reduce the risk of cancer and inhibit the growth of tumours.

10.3 SPIRULINA

Spirulina is the common name for human and animal food supplements produced from mainly two species of cyanobacteria: *Arthrospira platensis* and *Arthrospira maxima*. These, along with various other species of Arthrospira, were previously classed under the Spirulina genus. Now, it has been recognised that these cyanobacteria are a distinct genus but the name spirulina continues to be used. Spirulina is widely used as a whole food as well as a dietary supplement. It is also used as feed in poultry and aquaculture.

The main advantage of spirulina is its ability to grow in very hot and alkaline conditions. Since no other organism can survive such conditions, spirulina is obtained in the pure form, without contamination by other species. Therefore, it is claimed to be one of the cleanest and most sterile natural foods available today. The ability to withstand high temperatures also ensures that there is no loss of nutritional value during processing and storage.

Chemical constituents

Proteins

Spirulina is rich in proteins, containing between 55% and 77% by dry weight, depending on the source. It contains all the essential amino acids, although the proportion is less than in other complete proteins such as meat, eggs and milk. However, it is superior in quality to plant proteins.

Essential fatty acids

Spirulina is a rich source of linoleic acid, g-linolenic acid, a-linolenic acid, eicosapentaenoic acid and arachidonic acid.

Vitamins

Many vitamins of the B-complex group such as thiamine, riboflavin, pyridoxine, niacin, folic acid, ascorbic acid, and fat-soluble vitamins D and E are present in Spirulina.

Minerals

Spirulina contains various important minerals such as potassium, calcium, chromium, magnesium, manganese, iron, selenium, copper, phosphorus and zinc.

Photosynthetic pigments

Various photosynthetic pigments such as b-carotene, chlorophyll a, myxoxanthophyll, canthaxanthin, echinenone, hydroxy echinenone and phycobiliproteins are also present in spirulina.

Uses

- It has antioxidant property and the ability to build immune defence. Hence, it is used as a general tonic. Its utility in autoimmune diseases such as multiple sclerosis is under investigation.
- It has been shown to have relevant cytotoxic action in studies conducted on animals.
- It has natural anti-histaminic activity and hence, has significant anti-allergy properties.
- It contains large quantities of an antioxidant produced by the body called superoxide dismutase. Levels of this enzyme decline in old age and hence, spirulina is believed to be useful in slowing down ageing.
- It improves digestion when added to existing diets. It acts by suppressing the action of pathogenic bacteria while stimulating action of beneficial bacteria in the gastrointestinal tract.

10.3 SOYBEAN

Soybean is a seed of *Glycine max* and several other species of *Glycine soja, Glycine hispida* and *Soja hispida* belonging to the Leguminosae family.

About 150 varieties of soybeans are grown, but the yellow variety is the one generally used for nutritional purposes. Soybeans need processing to extract the oil and produce the soybean meal which is made up of 48% protein.

Uses

Soybean oil is used in cooking oils, sandwich spreads, salads and chocolate dressings, and also in medicines. Soybean meal is mainly used as feed for beef, dairy cattle and poultry, and, to a lesser extent, in human food products.

10.4 OMEGA-3 FATTY ACIDS

n-3 Fatty acids (popularly referred to as ω-3 fatty acids or omega-3 fatty acids) are a group of unsaturated fatty acids that have a final carbon–carbon double bond at the ω-position; that is, the third bond counting from the methyl-end of the fatty acid. These acids cannot be synthesized in the human body and are hence considered as essential fatty acids that need to be supplied through the diet. Fish such as tuna, salmon and halibut, along with algae, krill and purslane, and oil obtained from nuts such as hazelnuts, pecan nuts and walnuts are rich in omega-3 fatty acids. Flax and linseed are also good sources.

Uses

- Recent clinical research shows that omega-3 fatty acids are helpful in the treatment of cardiovascular disease. Those who consume greater quantities show higher concentrations of HDL cholesterol and low triglyceride levels.
- They are also considered useful in lowering blood pressure in hypertensive patients and preventing atherosclerosis.
- Supplements containing these acids have shown a marked ability to help reduce the tenderness, pain and inflammation of rheumatoid arthritis.
- Omega-3 fatty acids have also shown an ability to increase bone density in women aged above 65 with osteoporosis.
- They are also believed to be important for good mental health and people whose diets are deficient in this component are said to be at a higher risk of succumbing to depression. This is believed to be due to omega-3 fatty acids being a major component of the membranes of nerve cells and sufficient quantities are required to maintain their optimal functioning.

SUMMARY

- Nutraceuticals are foods with health benefits, including the prevention and treatment of disease.
- Food products used as nutraceuticals include antioxidants, prebiotics, probiotics, omega-3 fatty acids and certain dietary fibres.
- Garlic is an important compound used in traditional medicine for preventing many disorders.
- Spirulina is the common name for human and animal food supplements produced from cyanobacteria. It is used as an antioxidant, anti-cancer and anti-allergic agent and to boost the immune system.
- It has been found that omega-3 fatty acids may be helpful in treating a variety of health conditions, but mostly heart disease and associated problems.

Exercises

Long answers

1. Define, classify and describe nutraceuticals with examples.
2. Explain the uses of various nutraceuticals.

Short answers

3. Write a note on garlic.
4. What is spirulina? Describe its role as a nutraceutical compound.
5. Define the terms 'prebiotic' and 'probiotic'.

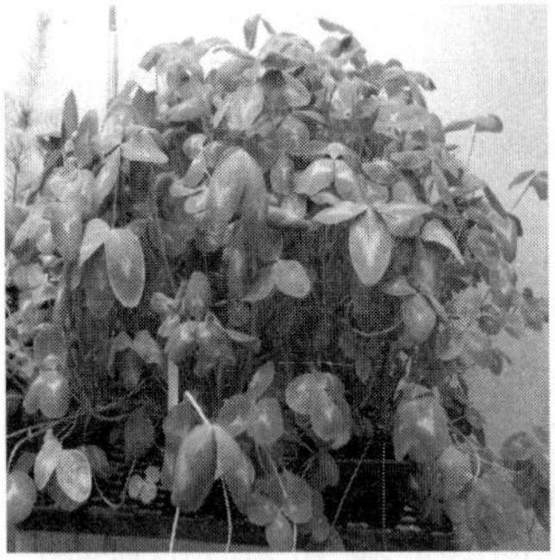

11

Polyploidy

In This Chapter, You Will Learn

- What is polyploidy
- The causes of polyploidy
- The different types of polyploidy and examples of polyploid crops
- The methods of inducing polyploidy
- The advantages of polyploidy
- The effects of polyploidy

The word 'ploidy' expresses the number of chromosome sets in a biological cell. The number of chromosomes in a germ cell or gamete is haploid (n). Somatic cells are produced from a combination of gametes from the male and female parent and therefore contain twice the number of chromosomes and are said to be diploid ($2n$). Other organisms, however, often have greater than two sets of chromosomes and such organisms are said to be 'polylpoid'. The word 'polyploidy' therefore is defined as the process of doubling of genomes that produce organisms with multiple chromosome sets. Polyploid plants can be triploid ($3n$), tetraploid ($4n$) and so on. Certain species of plants such as ferns, flowering plants such as Hibiscus, and wheat are more prone to polyploidy. Wheat occurs as diploid, tetraploid and hexaploid varieties. Polyploidy is a phenomenon that is common in plants, but rare in animals. Only a few animals such as salamanders, goldfish and salmon, exhibit polyploidy.

Polyploid plants are generally larger than the normal varieties. This property has been exploited to create bigger varieties of marigold flowers, watermelons and snapdragons.

Causes of polyploidy

Abnormality in cell division is the most significant cause of polyploidy. This commonly occurs due to an error during either meiosis or mitosis. During this process, there is a division of chromosomes that occurs without corresponding cell division. This is the reason why the use of drugs like colchicine that inhibit cell division can bring about polyploidy in the plants to which it is applied. Although polyploidy occurs in almost all somatic cells, the effects may sometimes be restricted to a particular type of tissue, when it is known as *endopolyploidy*.

Types of polyploidy

Polyploidy can be of two types: autopolyploidy and allopolyploidy.

Autopolyploids or autoploids

They are polyploids that arise from a single genotype (AAAA). In such cases, a common observation is the somatic doubling of zygote or vegetative cells that occur in the apical meristem. This doubling is almost always in even numbers.

Allopolyploids or alloploids

They are polyploids obtained from different genotypes (AABB). A common distinguishing character is the pairing of chromosomes that occurs during meiosis.

In other words, autoploids give rise to multivalent forms whereas alloploids form bivalent forms.

Applications of polyploidy

During commercial breeding of crops, it is always the tallest and fittest plants that are selected. This is because these plants have a greater chance of flourishing even under adverse conditions. This unintentional selection has led to crops being bred to polyploidy levels.

In certain cases, polyploidy is induced to overcome the obstacles posed by sterile hybrid species. For example, a hybridization of wheat, *Triticum turgidum,* and rye, *Secale cereal,* gives rise to the plant Triticale. This plant has the most desirable characteristics from both species but has the disadvantage of the first generation hybrids being sterile. In this case, formation of polyploidy can be used to make the hybrid fertile and help in further propagation.

In certain other cases, where sterility is a necessity, it makes sense to use polyploid crops which are sterile. This is the case with seedless fruit varieties; these fruits are rendered seedless by inducing polyploidy. Such crops can be further propagated using asexual methods such as grafting. Some examples of crops which have been improved by polyploidy are shown below:

Triploid: Apple, ginger, citrus, banana, water melon

Tetraploid: Macaroni wheat, potato, cotton, tobacco, cabbage, maize, peanuts

Hexaploid: Bread wheat, oat, triticale, chrysanthemum, kiwifruit

Octaploid: Sugar cane, strawberry, pansies and dahlia

Induction of polyploidy

Polyploidy occurs naturally in certain plant tissues due to the process of endo-replication. It can also be induced in plants when dividing cells are treated with an agent such as colchicine to prevent spindle formation. As a result of microtubule disruption, there is a failure in chromosome separation during mitosis. For example, onion cells on exposure to colchicine for a few days can give rise to more than 1,000 chromosomes.

When a newly-formed tetraploid plant is bred with an ancestral species in what is called as a *backcross*, it leads to the formation of triploid offspring which are sterile. This is because the assortment of chromosomes present does not allow the formation of gametes necessary for reproduction. A tetraploid plant can, however, breed with other tetraploid plants to form a new species.

Some of the methods for inducing polyploidy in various organisms are discussed here.

Cell generation

This method is useful in the case of bryophytes such as mosses. When the diploid sporophytes are cut off and stored under moist conditions, polyploidy is induced. The cells located at the incised ends regenerate threads that are true protonema and this leads to the production of diploid gametophytes instead of the usual haploid ones.

Physical agents

Certain physical conditions are capable of inducing polyploidy in plants:

Temperature shocks Sudden, extreme changes in temperature can increase the number of polyploid cells produced.

Centrifugation When plant seedlings are centrifuged, it leads to the production of polyploid cells. In Nicotiana, for instance, polyploidy has been successfully induced through the use of this method.

X-rays Various radioactive agents such as radium and radiation such as x-rays have shown promising results in inducing polyploidy in diploid plant cells.

Chemical agents

Although colchicine is the most commonly used chemical agent, various other compounds such as chloral hydrate, ethyl and mercuric chloride, acenaphthene, sulfanilamide, veratrine and hexachlorocyclohexane have been reported with significant ability to induce polyploidy in plants when applied to dividing diploid cells. They are believed to act by causing a disturbance of mitotic spindle formation, which in turn leads to a non-segregation of chromosomes that have already duplicated. This, in turn causes a conversion of the diploid cells to tetraploid cells, which can be further converted into different levels of polyploidy.

Advantages of polyploidy

- *Polyploid offspring are healthier than both the diploid parents.* This can be due to the enforced pairing between homologous chromosomes that prevents the parent cell genomes from combining. Thus, heterozygosity is maintained and this, in turn, prevents the build-up of recessive mutations in later generation genomes, leading to retention of hybrid vigour.
- *Polyploidy also leads to gene redundancy* because of multiple copies of the gene in the polyploid offspring. This implies that the offspring are protected from the damaging effects of any recessive mutations that may occur. This effect can be especially important in conditions where there is inbreeding of smaller, isolated populations.
- *Gene redundancy also leads to another benefit of gene function diversification over time.* Due to this, the excess gene copies which do not perform any role in normal functioning of the organism will often be used for different roles in evolutionary selection.
- The effect of polyploidy on sexual character bestows various advantages in improving selectivity during breeding. Polyploidy promotes the onset of reproduction by asexual methods besides allowing self-fertilization.

Effects of polyploidy

Morphological changes

Polyploidy can cause changes in the morphological characteristics of the plants, such as, increase in the size of flowers and fruits. In case of flowers, those with larger size and with larger and more number of pollen grains and stomata are produced. Occasionally, as in the case of Lobelia, smaller plants may also be produced.

Chemical changes

There are major chemical changes as a result of polyploidy in plants. There is a change in not just the total content of certain secondary metabolites, but also an alteration of their relative proportions. Examples of changes in chemical content on polyploidy are shown in Table 11.1.

Table 11.1 Chemical changes on polyploidy

Name of the drug	Active constituent	Percentage content in $2n$	Percentage content in $4n$
Atropa belladona	Hyoscine, dry weight	0.2%	68% increase over $2n$
Cinchona succirubra	Quinine, dry weight	0.53%	1.12%

Proportion of constituents

Polyploidy often causes an alteration in the proportion of individual constituents. For example, *Digitalis lanata* when subjected to polyploidy exhibits a selective increase in lanatoside content without any significant change in the proportions of other glycosides.

SUMMARY

- Polyploidy is the process of doubling the genome. It gives rise to organisms with multiple sets of chromosomes.
- Polyploidy can arise from spontaneous duplication of somatic chromosomes or as a result of non-disjunction of the homologous chromosomes during meiosis resulting in diploid gametes. It can also be artificially induced by treatment with drugs, such as colchicine.
- Polyploidy can be of two types: autopolyploidy and allopolyploidy.
- Polyploid plants have several advantages such as larger size and the ability to overcome sterility of hybrid species. They have been used to produce seedless varieties of fruits.
- Polyploidy can also help in increasing the concentration of individual constituents, in particular, plants like Digitalis.

Exercises

Short answers

1. Define polyploidy.
2. What are the different methods by which polyploidy can occur?
3. What are the effects of polyploidy?
4. What is endo-replication?
5. What are the different chemicals used for inducing polyploidy?
6. Give some examples of plants obtained by polyploidy.
7. Define the terms autopolyploidy and allopolyploidy.

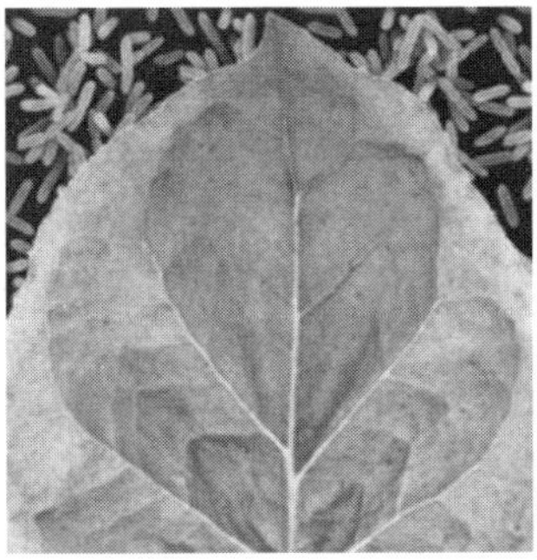

12

Plant Biotechnology

In This Chapter, You Will Learn

- What is biotechnology
- The applications of plant biotechnology
- The applications of plant tissue culture
- What is biotransformation and what are secondary metabolites

Plant biotechnology began with the use of microorganisms for fermentation. The history of this field consists of three phases, each characterized by a milestone:

1. In the 1920s, *Clostridium acetobutylicum* was used to convert starch into butanol and acetone.
2. In the 1940s, penicillin was produced from cultures of *Penicillium notatum.*
3. In recent times, the principles of biotechnology have been adopted in developing techniques such as recombinant DNA technology.

Definition

Biotechnology is the product of interaction between the science of biology and technology. The older concept of biotechnology involved processes such as fermentation by microorganisms, formation of curd and cheese from milk, vinegar from molasses, the production of antibiotics from fungi, and the processes of baking and brewing. Modern biotechnology deals with recombinant DNA, polymerase chain reaction (PCR), cell culture and fusion and bio-processing.

Some of the definitions proposed for biotechnology include:

1. *British biotechnologists*: The application of biological organisms, systems or processes to manufacturing and service industries.

2. *European Federation of Biotechnology*: Integrated use of biochemistry, microbiology, and the engineering sciences in order to achieve technological (industrial) application of the capabilities of microorganisms, cultured tissue cells and parts thereof.
3. *Japanese biotechnologists*: A technology using biological phenomena for copying and manufacturing various kinds of useful substances.
4. *US National Science Foundation*: This is often considered the briefest, yet most comprehensive definition: Biotechnology is the controlled use of biological agents, such as microorganisms or cellular components, for beneficial use.
5. *UN Convention on Biodiversity*: Biotechnology means any technological application that uses biological systems, living organisms, or derivatives thereof, to make or modify products or processes for specific use.

Pharmacobiotechnology

Robbers et al coined this term in 1996. It refers to the wide application of biotechnology to the development of pharmaceuticals or pharmaceutically active substances.

Table 12.1 Modern products developed by pharmacobiotechnology

Product / Brand	Used in
Actimmune	Chronic granulomatous disease
Betaseron	Relapsing, remitting, multiple sclerosis
Epogen	Anaemia associated with chronic renal failure
KoGenate	Haemophilia A
Leupine	Autologous bone marrow transplantation
Oncoscint Cr/Ov	Detection, staging and follow up of colorectal and ovarian cancer
Proleukin	Renal cell carcinoma

12.1 SCOPE OF BIOTECHNOLOGY

- Tissue culture techniques can be used with microorganisms or plant and animal cells (or protoplasts in case of plants), or tissues and organs in artificial media. Cultured microorganisms can be used for recombinant DNA technology. Plant cells and tissues are used in wide-ranging genetic manipulations such as haploid breeding, production of artificial seeds and production of useful transgenic plants.
- Gene technology—also called genetic engineering—is used by most companies manufacturing biotechnology products. It involves recombinant DNA and gene cloning, and recently, PCR.
- The use of hybridoma and monoclonal antibodies is a rapidly growing field.

Enzyme conjugated antibodies are used for the detection of viruses by ELISA tests. Immunotoxins are also being produced by gene fusion to deliver drugs to kill tumour cells directly to the target sites using specific antibodies.

- In medicine, bacterially synthesized drugs such as insulin and interferon are already in use. Vaccines for immunization, DNA probes and monoclonal antibodies for diagnosis of various diseases, human growth hormone and other pharmaceutical drugs are also being released. DNA fingerprinting and auto-antibody fingerprinting techniques are proving a great boon in forensic medicine for the identification of criminals.
- Protein (or enzyme) engineering has been used for the production of superior enzymes and storage proteins. This process involves the initial preparation of a computer-aided model of a protein to perform a specific function, followed by the synthesis of a gene to produce the desired protein as predicted by the genetic code. Another important application is in immobilized enzyme systems that allow for the production of a variety of substances such as high-fructose corn syrup using an immobilized enzyme glucose isomerase.
- Metabolic engineering involves the use of principles of biotechnology to manipulate metabolic pathways in such a manner that there is overproduction of certain metabolites or heterologous genes and an introduction of some regulatory elements.
- In agriculture, the various applications of biotechnology include:
    - Plant cell, tissue and organ culture
    - Genetic engineering, which is a regeneration of plants, leading to the production of transgenic plants with desirable traits like disease resistance, insect resistance, and herbicide resistance. It can also be used to enhance other qualities such as photosynthetic efficiency, nitrogen fixing ability, improved storage proteins, hybrid crops, etc.
    - Somatic hybridization between sexually incompatible species is possible due to a transfer of desirable traits from wild/unrelated crop species to our crop plants.
    - Transgenic animals have been produced in species of mice, pig, goat, hen and cow. Some of these may ultimately be used as 'bioreactors' to produce drugs from their milk, blood or urine, through a process called 'molecular farming'.
- Industrial microbiology uses biotechnology for the production of better quality and increased quantities of pharmaceutical drugs and chemicals.
- Environmental applications of biotechnology make it possible to deal with environmental problems such as pollution control, restoration of degraded land and conservation of biodiversity. In recent times, microorganisms have been developed for use as biopesticides, biofertilizers and biosensors to help in recovery of metals, cleaning spilled oils, and for biomonitoring in industries.

12.2 TISSUE CULTURE

Broadly speaking, the term tissue culture is used to refer to the growth of tissues/cells separate from the organism from which they are derived. Tissue culture commonly refers to the culture of both animal cells and tissues; to indicate the tissue culture of plants, it is apt to use the more specific term 'plant tissue culture'.

Tissue culture is a process in which small pieces of living tissue called 'explants' are isolated from an organism and grown aseptically for an indefinite period of time on a defined nutrient medium. A wide range of material can be used as explants such as seedlings and organs, single cells and protoplasts. Meristematic cells in plants proliferate rapidly and hence, using meristematic tissue ensures better success with tissue culture. This is typically facilitated by use of a liquid, semi-solid, or solid growth media, such as broth or agar.

TOTIPOTENCY

For many years, we have known that plant material is capable of growth and division in vitro. This property is referred to as 'totipotency'. It means a single cell has the potential to regenerate into the whole organism. The multiplication of a single cell into complex multicellular tissues and organs is a natural progression in plants, which occurs through a series of highly coordinated processes. The degree to which a plant undergoes differentiation and maturation is dependent on the constitution of inherited genes as well as the provision made for supplying the right conditions during the process of mitotic cell division.

Cell division takes place mainly due to the activity of apical meristem which is responsible for the growth and differentiation of cells. The activity of the meristems is controlled by certain genetic/environmental control mechanisms. For totipotency to be possible, it is vital that the new somatic cells derived from the meristem retain their functional and conserved DNA during the process of differentiation. The mechanism involved in this gene differentiation should retain the property of gene expression, without causing any permanent modifications in the genome during differentiation.

Advantages of plant tissue culture

Plant tissue culture is widely used to propagate plants under sterile conditions, often to produce clones of a plant. This method proffers the following advantages over traditional methods of propagation.

1. It is possible to produce a large number of clones that produce good flowers or fruits or have other desirable traits from a single explant.
2. The selection of desirable traits is possible, thus reducing the need for field trials.
3. The time required for growth is less than that required for traditional methods.

4. This technique is especially beneficial for species that have a long generation time, low level of seed production, or exhibit a lack of seed germination. It allows the production of plants from seeds that do not generally germinate or grow easily, such as, orchids and nepenthes.
5. The seasonal limitations on germination can be overcome.
6. The pollen and cell collections can be preserved using certain storage methods, so that plants can be propagated from these reserves whenever required (like a seed bank).
7. Stock can be carefully selected and sterile techniques that help reduce or eliminate plant diseases can be used.
8. The plants that are produced within sterile containers can be moved more conveniently, with less risk of transmitting diseases, pests and pathogens, which facilitates their international exchange.
9. A large number of viable plants can be easily stored in a small space.

Applications of plant tissue culture

Plant tissue culture is used widely for scientific and commercial applications.

- Plant breeders use tissue culture for screening cells for characteristics such as resistance to insecticides and herbicides.
- Tissue culture can be used to grow cultures in bioreactor vessels to produce biopharmaceuticals.
- Micropropagation is of great value in floriculture and forestry. It is also useful in conservation of endangered plant species.
- Techniques such as meristem tip culture help in the formation of uncontaminated plant material using virus-infested stock, as in the case of potatoes and some fruits.
- Tissue culture can help in crossing species through the process of protoplast fusion to generate a new variety.
- Cross-pollination followed by tissue culture results in the preservation of embryos that otherwise generally do not survive. This process is known as embryo rescue.
- Tissue culture has been used for the production of dihaploid plants to give rapid breeding of homozygous lines. This involves treatment with agents such as colchicine to cause doubling of chromosome number.

Equipment required for a plant tissue culture laboratory

Essential facilities that a tissue culture laboratory should have are as follows:

- *Incubator* with forced air circulation, with a temperature control of ± 0.5°C and safety thermostat. Temperature recommended for most tissue culture studies is

36.5°C. The incubators are generally made of stainless steel (SS) or anodized aluminium and should be corrosion resistant.

- *Autoclave* that can generate a pressure of 1 atmosphere or 15 pounds per square inch (psi). The simplest form of an autoclave is a pressure cooker.
- *Refrigerators and freezers* to store reagents, stock solutions and chemicals. A domestic refrigerator of larger capacity without an ice box can be used for this purpose. The ice box should be removed to avoid defrosting.
- *Microscopes* to study morphological changes in cultures. This is important because morphological change in the culture medium can indicate deterioration of the culture. The stage of the microscope should be large enough to accommodate large roller bottles in specific cases. Provision should be made for attachment of a camera to enable the photography of living cultures.
- *Washing equipment* to wash glassware, large aspirators, pipettes, etc. There should also be deep soaking baths or washing sinks constructed of stainless steel or polypropylene to allow manual washing and rinsing of all types of glassware, except pipettes. Washing sinks should be fitted with 4 taps— single cold water, combined cold/hot water, cold hose connection for rinsing device and non-metallic tap for de-ionized (DI) water. For pipette washing, siphon type pipette washers are used.
- *Dry heat sterilization oven* for sterilization of pipettes and other glassware. This is important to avoid the possibility of chemical contamination from steam condensate or corrosion of pipette cans.
- *Water purification system* to provide pure water. De-ionized water is suitable for rinsing glassware but higher purity water is needed for the preparation of all the media and reagents. Reverse osmosis filtration, de-ionization and millipore filtration are used. Sometimes, distillation is preferred instead of reverse osmosis as it gives sterile water.
- *Centrifuge* for routine laboratory work. A small bench top centrifuge with proportionally controlled braking is sufficient for most purposes.
- *Shakers* to agitate suspension cultures. A rotary shaker or reciprocal shaker is needed for suspension cultures.
- *Shelves* for storage of glassware. These should be constructed of rigid wire mesh to allow maximum air movement and minimum shading in the culture room.
- *Culture room/cabinet* Culture rooms maintained under different temperatures or cabinet-type incubators are needed to cultivate the plant cells. Temperature and light intensity as well as the duration of lighting in the rooms/cabinet need to be controlled under optimal conditions.
- *Laminar air flow (LAF) cabinet* This is a sterile chamber for carrying out processes such as the transfer of tissue into media in glass vials or Erlenmeyer flasks. A glow box is the simplest transfer cabin filled with a germicidal tube and can be used in place of a LAF cabinet for inoculation.

- *Other requirements* include
  - ample space for the storage of chemicals, glassware, culture containers, etc., under dust-free conditions
  - equipment such as a hot plate, stirrer, pH meter, semi-microbalances, Bunsen burners with gas cylinders
  - vacuum and sources of compressed air
  - space for media preparation and aseptic transfer
  - shelves to maintain cultures

Other useful equipment in a tissue culture laboratory include cell counters, vacuum pumps, carbon dioxide incubator, osmometer, densitometer, phase contrast and fluorescent microscope, magnetic stirrer, separate sterilizing and drying oven, glassware washing machine, colony counter and a high-capacity centrifuge.

A plant tissue culture laboratory should have good work flow, with orderly movement of supplies, people, cultures and finished products. There should be a minimum number of entry points in order to keep air-borne contaminants at low levels. There should be clearly designated 'clean rooms' with a high-efficiency particulate air (HEPA) filter allowing purified air under positive pressure.

Facilities in a plant tissue culture laboratory

In a plant tissue culture laboratory, separate areas are required for preparation and storage of media, transfer, culture, cold storage, locker and shipping. Each of these is explained below.

Media preparation

This area should contain many counters, shelves, pH meter, autoclaves, media dispersing equipment and a dishwashing area. Storage space should be provided for empty culture vessels. Autoclaves create heat load. Hence, they should be placed on the side of the exterior wall with good, clean ventilation.

Media storage

This area is needed for cooling and storage of dispersed media. It is generally combined with media preparation room or is in a section of the transfer room.

Transfer room

It the heart of the plant tissue culture laboratory. It should be provided with a LAF hood where most of the culture initiation and sub-culturing is performed. Other processes such as culture re-plantation, transfer or re-initiation cultures in a clean media, and the harvesting of 'ripe' cultures are also performed here. The tools used are sterilized at the hood using alcohol or glass head sterilizers and flame. This room should be provided with an efficient air-conditioning system to compensate for the heat load generated by hood, sterilizers and workers.

Culture room

This is the largest area of the lab. Here, cultures are incubated on shelves under specific conditions of temperature and light. The quality and quantity of light is an important factor that influences the success of tissue culture. Generally, high output, cool, white and fluorescent lighting is preferred, because higher intensities may cause a problem of heat control. The temperature conditions are often crop specific, but range from 18–20°C. Good movement of air is critical in equalizing the temperature throughout the culture room.

Cold storage

This area may not be required as a separate unit in smaller laboratories, but is an essential component of commercial tissue culture labs. Cold storage (temperature of 2–4 °C) is used to maintain stock blocks in culture for plants, to provide chilling requirements for crops such as apples and pears.

Locker room

This is the area where employees working in the tissue culture laboratory change into appropriate clothing for working in the lab.

Shipping area

This is the place from where the harvested, boxed or packed ripe product is shipped.

Culture media

Media used in tissue culture should be prepared with the perfect balance of nutritional and hormonal requirements of the entire plant. Culture media ingredients can be of two types:

- Components that are indispensable for the growth of most cell cultures
- Components that are not required, but are beneficial or occasionally necessary for the growth of specific cells in a particular condition

Components of nearly all plant culture media can be divided into six groups:

- Major inorganic nutrients
- Trace elements
- Iron source
- Vitamins
- Carbon source
- Plant growth regulators

Major inorganic nutrients

These nutrients are also called macronutrients or macroelements. They include nitrogen, phosphorus, potassium, calcium, magnesium and sulphur. These are required at milligram levels. Generally, the level of ammonium needed is less than that of nitrate. It has been found that organic nitrogen (obtained from amino acids such as proline and glutamine) is more beneficial in enhancing somatic embryogenesis and organogenesis in certain species than inorganic nitrogen. Calcium is important for the organization of the middle lamella of the cell wall, magnesium for the synthesis of chlorophyll and phosphorus for providing an important structural element of DNA and RNA, the cell membrane and ATP.

Trace elements

These are required in very small quantities, and yet, the media lacking these do not support healthy and wholesome growth. Plants which are grown on such media show deficiency symptoms. Boron, manganese, copper, molybdenum, chloride, nickel, aluminium, cobalt, iodine, iron and sodium are a few of the important trace elements. In general, plants thrive on 17 elements, of which four—C, H, O, N—are derived from the atmosphere and the remaining 13 are obtained from the soil. Absence of these essential elements in the medium leads to various deficiency symptoms in the callus cultures, such as, the occurrence of pigmentation, absence of vessels and presence of narrow cambial zone, cellular hypertrophy and symptoms of chlorosis.

Iron source

Culture media often contain iron in the form of ferric sulphate but a chelated iron source such as Fe-EDTA is preferred because it remains stable longer and does not get depleted easily. Instead of the common salts of iron, Sequesterene 330 Fe is used in certain media. Iron is required for synthesis of chlorophyll as well as in many oxidation and reduction reactions.

Vitamins

Many plants synthesize vitamins in trace quantities and therefore, their addition to culture media may not be necessary unless otherwise specified. They are required for the healthy growth of tissue in the culture media. Vitamin B-complex plays a catalytic role in cell metabolism. Of all these vitamins, only thiamine may be required for most tissue cultures. Vitamin C in high concentrations behaves as an antioxidant. Folic acid, riboflavine, PABA, Vitamin B12 and biotin are sometimes added in special cases, but their exact role is not yet established.

Carbon source

Most tissue cultures are heterotrophic and therefore, various carbohydrates are used as a carbon source in culture media. Sucrose is the most preferred and necessary component in the culture medium, because it serves as the main osmoticum. Besides, it helps in rapid growth and organogenesis. It also has a role in enhancing the ability of the cells to use ammonium and nitrate ions. The only disadvantage of using sucrose is the possibility of degradation when the medium is autoclaved. This causes formation of sugar acids, which may react with other components in the medium.

Other carbohydrates such as glucose, fructose, pentoses, sugar alcohol and glycols may also be employed.

Plant growth regulators

The growth and development of higher plant tissues in vitro is controlled by endogenous plant growth regulators. Five groups of regulators are commonly used:

- Auxins
- Cytokinins
- Gibberellins
- Unsaturated hydrocarbon gases
- Growth inhibitors

AUXINS They are found in actively growing tissues such as stem and root apices. Indole acetic acid (IAA) is a naturally occurring auxin (Fig. 12.1 a). Synthetic auxins include indole butyric acid (IBA), naphthalene acetic acid (NAA), 2,4-dichlorophenoxy acetic acid (2,4-D), *p*-chlorophenoxy acetic acid (p-CPA) and trichlorophenoxy acetic acid (2,4,5-T) (Fig. 12.1 b). They are generally used in the range of 0.1–10 mg/l in plant tissue culture media.

Auxins perform the following functions:

- Initiate cell division and stimulate shoot growth but inhibit root growth
- Regulate differentiation of the vascular system and apical dominance
- Delay senescence
- Promote flowering, fruit setting and ripening
- IBA and NAA are used for promoting root formation and can be applied along with cytokinins for shoot proliferation
- 2,4-D and 2, 4, 5-T cause induction and growth of callus

CYTOKININS They are mostly produced in the roots. An important degradation product of DNA, also found in fresh nucleic acid preparations after autoclaving, is 6-furfuryl aminopurine (Fig. 12.2). It causes significant proliferation of cells. The first synthetic analogue of kinetin, 6-benzyl aminopurine, also gives a similar effect. Cytokinins, in concentrations of 40–80 mg/l, are used in most plant regeneration studies. They can induce morphogenesis and in higher concentrations, cause speedy multiplication of

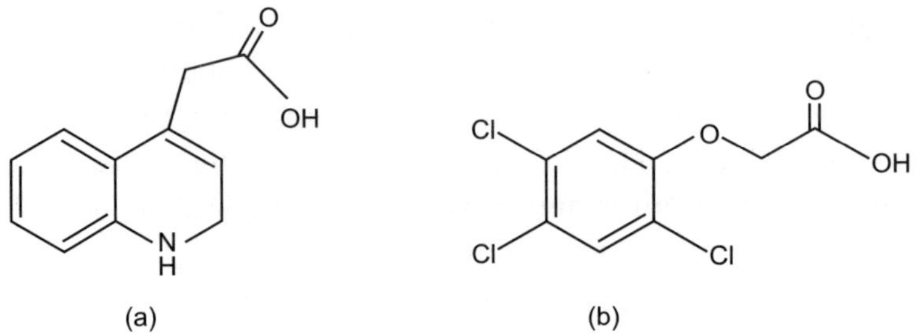

Fig. 12.1 (a) Auxins and (b) Trichlorophenoxy acetic acid (2,4,5-T)

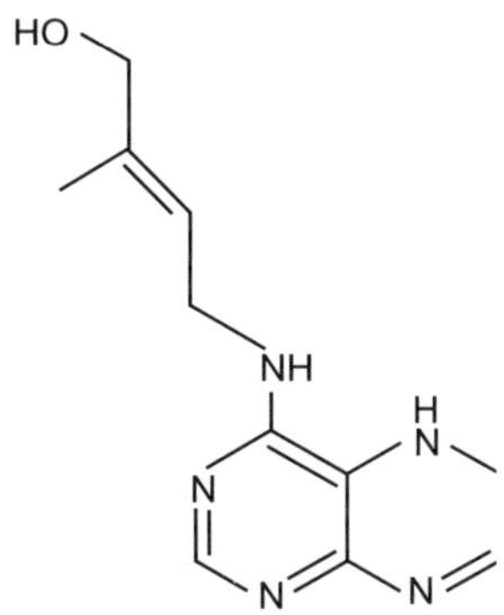

Fig. 12.2 Cytokinins

shoots, axillary/adventitious buds or meristems. The use of these compounds inhibits rooting. It has been observed that synthetic auxins work synergistically with cytokinins and do not evoke any response if used alone.

Gibberellins: They are produced in leaves and collect in the immature fruits and seeds. There are 84 well-known gibberellins (Fig. 12.3); of these, GA3 is mainly used on adventive embryos formed in culture for inducing plantlet formation. Gibberellins have the following effects:

- Hyperelongation of stems when applied to dwarf plants
- Stimulate flowering
- Elongation of internode and division of sub-apical cell
- Induction of parthenocarpy

Ethylene It is a gaseous hormone synthesized in fungi, bacteria and in cultured cells (Fig. 12.4). It has an important action on various metabolic processes and the developmental process of higher plants. Auxins tend to increase the production of ethylene.

Abscisic acid (ABA) This compound, similar in structure to carotenoids, occurs as a natural product in plant tissue. Chemically, it is a sesquiterpene (Fig. 12.5).

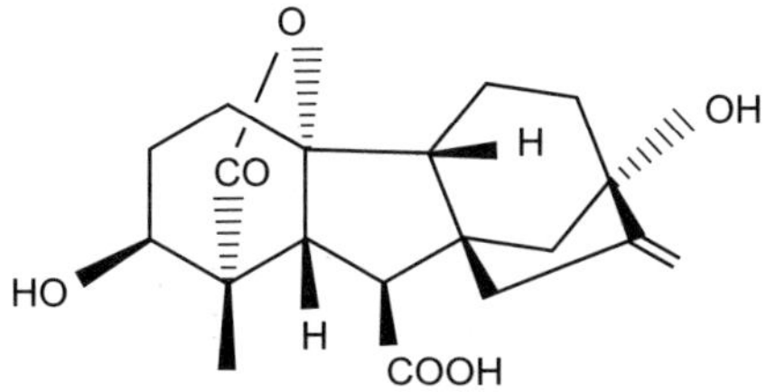

Fig. 12.3 Gibberellins

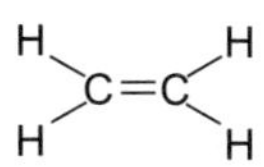

Fig.12.4 Ethylene

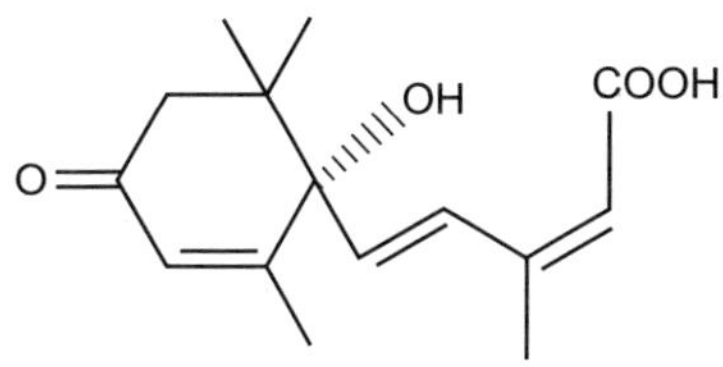

Fig. 12.5 Abscisic acid

It is believed that low ABA levels may stimulate somatic embryogenesis. It has the following effects:

- Increases the rate of abscission of leaves
- Extends dormancy of buds
- Retards germination and bud development

Other media substances

Agar It is used in plant tissue culture media as it helps to provide a surface that supports culture growth; but, it is not a nutrient. Generally, a 0.6%–0.8% agar solution is used as a gelling agent. This is necessary; if a liquid medium is used, the tissue sinks and dies due to lack of oxygen. However, it is important to avoid adding excess of agar as it can lead to hardening of the medium which in turn affects the ability of the culture to take up nutrients from it. The alternative is to provide regular aeration to liquid culture media by gentle agitation or by bubbling sterile air through the culture vessel.

Natural extracts Substances like coconut milk, fruit juice (tomato, banana), yeast extract, malt extract and casein hydrolysate help promote tissue growth. Amino acids such as arginine, asparagine, cystein HCl and glutamine are also added.

Activated charcoal When added as a fine powder, it helps to adsorb toxic tissue exudates which can inhibit growth of the tissue if left within the medium.

Other factors influencing growth

Light

Light has culture-inducing properties and is also required for the growth of plant tissues. The optimum light intensity varies between species.

Temperature

Temperature should be maintained within the range of 25–27°C, since this is the most suitable for callus growth. However, during the dark phase of callus differentiation, lower temperatures are better.

pH

The pH of the medium is generally adjusted to between 5.6 and 6.0 before autoclaving. This is important because a medium that is highly acidic or alkaline will have a significant negative effect on the uptake of nutrients by culture cells.

Relative humidity

Relative humidity (RH) of the rooms where culture incubation and growth take place should be maintained between 70%–75%. It has been found that low RH around 50%–55% leads to a dehydration of the medium, whereas higher RH of 85%–90% often encourages microbial growth that will ultimately contaminate both the medium and culture.

Table 12.2 Composition of Murashige and Skoog (MS) culture medium

Ingredient	Amount (mg/l)
Sucrose	30000
NH_4NO_3	1650
KNO_3	1900
$CaCl_2.2H_2O$	440
$MgSO_4.7H_2O$	370
KH_2PO_4	170
$FeSO_4.4H_2O$	27.8
Na_2EDTA	37.8
$MnSO_4.4H_2O$	22.3
$ZnSO_4.7H_2O$	8.6
H_2SO_3	6.2
KI	0.83
$NaHPO_4.2H_2O$	0.25
$CoCl_2.6H_2O$	0.025
Myo. inositol	100
Glycine	2.0
Kinetin (a cytokinetic)	0.04–10.0
Indole acetic acid	1.0–30.0

Media formulations

The most commonly used medium is the Murashige and Skoog (MS) medium (Table 12.2) which was formulated for the culture of tobacco explants. However, this medium has a very high salt content. This has been modified in White's medium. Another medium used is Gamborg's B5 medium made for soybean callus culture, which contains a higher proportion of nitrates compared to ammonium ions.

The composition of the medium plays a major role in determining the morphological characteristics of tissues that arise from the initial explants. This is especially true with regard to the plant hormones and the nitrogen source (nitrate versus ammonium salts or amino acids). It has been demonstrated that high levels of auxin often cause a rapid proliferation of roots, whereas an excess of cytokinin promotes shoot generation. The best growth of callus is observed when there is a balance in the concentrations of both auxin and cytokinin.

Media preparation

Earlier, media were prepared by weighing out and dissolving the individual ingredients in water. Currently, media are available in dry powder form which has to be dissolved in distilled water. Agar and sugar need to be added at this stage and the final volume is made up to the desired level using distilled water. After adjusting the pH to between 5.0 and 6.0, the medium is sterilized by autoclaving and then poured into the culture vessels, plugged with non-adsorbent cotton wool wrapped in cheese cloth. These vessels are stored in baskets, covered with aluminium foil and sterilized by autoclaving at 121°C for 15 minutes. If plastic culture vials are used, they cannot be autoclaved and hence, the medium is autoclaved in 250- or 500-ml flasks, cooled to 60°C and poured into the culture vials under aseptic conditions. Culture vessels are stored at 4°C and used whenever needed.

Choice of explant

Many morphological plant parts and tissues can be used as explants to initiate growth of cultures. Based on work with tobacco plants, there are claims that any part of a plant will yield totipotent explants. However, this is not true in all cases, as plant organs differ in their rates of growth and regeneration. This is because various cells in the plant exist in different stages of the cell cycle. Besides, they also differ in their ability to transport growth regulators, and in their capacity for metabolism. Some plant parts show an inability to grow in vitro. Selecting the right explants is important because this determines if the plantlets that develop will be haploid or diploid. Moreover, the origin of the explants is crucial in deciding the microbial pre-load of the culture, and affects the amount of time and effort involved in the tissue culture process.

Parts which include the meristematic ends of plants such as the stem tip, auxiliary bud tip and root tip make for good explants. Not only do these tissues have rapid and high rates of cell division, they also show an ability to produce and concentrate auxins and cytokinins in the required proportions. However, care has to be exercised in selecting the best explant material. For example, the root tip is a problematic tissue to work with because it is highly contaminated with soil microflora tightly bound to the root systems within the soil. During removal of this soil and consequently the microbes, there is a danger of injuring the root parts, which lays the foundation for further microbial contamination. Microbial contamination in turn leads to a destruction of the explant's growth potential. Although aerial explants such as the tip of the stem and bud are also likely to be contaminated with microflora, disinfecting these parts is easier through a simple surface sterilization method. They are also easier to locate because of visual discrepancies such as decolourization or necrosis of the plant part.

The problem of contamination can be avoided by using explants from seedlings. Surface sterilized seeds can be grown aseptically to yield seedlings, and these can be used to initiate tissue cultures. Since seeds are impermeable to penetration by surface sterilizing agents, even harsh agents such as hypochlorite can be used, which is not a viable option with other explants.

Preparation of explant

Excised plant parts to be used as explants should be sterilized using chemical agents before they are subdivided and used in inoculation. The simplest way of doing this is to wash the plant part under running tap water for about one hour, followed by surface sterilization using calcium or sodium hypochlorite solutions. Following this, the plant parts should be washed and rinsed in sterile, double-distilled water.

Sterilizing agents

Bleaching powder ($CaOCl_2$) has about 37%–44% of chlorine content. An aqueous solution of bleaching powder is one of the best sterilizing agents. The explant material should be immersed in this for 20 minutes with occasional shaking to dislodge contaminants. Higher concentrations will be required when woody explants are used, or in the case of explants infested with heavy microbial loads.

A 0.5%–2% solution of sodium hypochlorite is generally used with most tissues. This is the preferred method in cases where the explants are known to have moderate to low levels of bacterial contamination. Treatment with either of these, calcium or sodium hypochlorite, does not show any inhibition in the growth characteristics of the tissue.

Other agents such as mercuric chloride, hydrogen peroxide, bromine water, ethyl alcohol, silver nitrate, and antibiotics like Penicillin G, oxytetracycline and rifampicin can also be used as sterilizing agents.

When fruits and pods are used to initiate growth, they are first disinfected by dipping into a 70%–80% ethanol solution and subjected to flaming. Following this, the fruit or pod is split open to obtain seeds. The seeds are collected in sterile petri plates containing a cotton pad and filter paper.

Measurement of growth parameters

The growth of any tissue, callus or cell suspension culture is monitored by observing the increase in fresh or dry weight of cells or the increase in cell number. Other parameters such as packed cell volume, protein and DNA content, mitotic index, cell viability and so on may also be used to estimate the growth occurring in the cultures.

Stages in tissue culture

When explants from differentiated tissue are cultured by growing them on a nutrient medium, the meristematic state is first attained by the non-dividing, quiescent cells. This phenomenon, in which the mature cells revert to the immature meristematic state, causes the formation of a callus by the process of de-differentiation. These callus cells are capable of giving rise to an entire plant through the process called re-differentiation.

Plant cells possess this characteristic property of de-differentiation and re-differentiation which leads to cellular totipotency. This property is found only in plant cells. In other words, a single plant cell can give rise to a whole plant, but animal cells do not have this property. Animal cells lose their capacity to regenerate after undergoing differentiation.

Before cells undergo re-differentiation, they have to pass through a callus phase, although in certain rare cases, the de-differentiated cells produce whole plants directly without passing through the intermediate callus phase.

Cytodifferentiation

Callus cells in the undifferentiated state are all parenchymatous in nature. Therefore, for regeneration of the entire plant, these cells need to differentiate into a variety of cells. This process is mainly influenced by the presence of growth regulators such as auxins, with cytokinins and gibberellins aiding the process of differentiation into xylem tissue. At low concentrations (0.5 mg/l), auxins have been shown to stimulate xylem formation and there is an inverse relationship between auxin concentration and the degree of xylem differentiation. This effect of auxin is dependent on the presence of sugar.

Organogenic differentiation

For regeneration of a whole plant from a callus mass, mere cytodifferentiation is not sufficient; it requires differentiation which can lead to organogenesis (that is, formation of stem, roots and flowers). This can occur in two ways: shoot bud differentiation and somatic embryogenesis.

Growth profile of single cell culture

The different stages of growth are as follows:

1. *Lag phase*: Here, the cells are exposed to a fresh medium. Hence, they start to divide and the tissue shows slow growth.
2. *Exponential phase*: This phase is characterized by a rapid multiplication of cells, with the onset of this phase varying according to the cell and its nutrient regime. This phase is usually of short duration and lasts for 3–4 generations.
3. *Linear phase*: In this stage, growth follows a linear pattern.
4. *Progressive deceleration phase*: During this phase, there is a decrease in the rate of cell division as the culture ages.
5. *Stationary phase*: This is the phase when there is no further growth of cells and the rate of cell formation equals the rate of cellular death.
6. *Senescent phase*: During this last phase of cell culture, cells die due to the non-availability of nutrients.

Growth profile of callus culture

The different stages of growth in callus culture are:

1. *Lag phase*: After inoculation of the explant into the nutrient media, there is an initial lag period when the cells do not show any growth but begin adapting to the new nutritional environmental conditions.
2. *Exponential phase*: Here, the cells multiply rapidly and consume nutrients from the medium, leading to a depletion in the levels of these ingredients.
3. *Decline phase*: Depletion of nutrients is responsible for starvation of some cells which in turn causes a decline in the growth of callus tissue.
4. *Stationary phase*: From this stage onwards, there is no evidence of growth, and sub-culturing of the cells is necessary to induce further growth and development.

The various techniques for measuring the growth of cultures are:

- Cell number
- Packed cell volume
- Fresh and dry weights
- Nutrient uptake studies
- Cell viability measurements such as cytoplasmic streaming, membrane integrity measurement and biochemical activity measurement

Techniques of plant tissue culture

Plant tissue culture techniques include the following methods:

Embryo culture In this method, embryo cells are cultivated on agar media and further allowed to grow into plants.

Organ culture Certain organs such as the meristem tip are excised from plants and used in the process of generating the entire plant.

Callus culture or Static culture This type of culture involves situations where some tissues are excised from an adult plant. When these tissues are grown in a culture medium, they form a structure called callus. It serves as the starting point to develop new tissue.

Plant cell culture Such cultures involve the dissociation of cells into a single-cell suspension, which can be used for the further generation of new plants.

The most important one is the cell suspension culture, because it permits the isolation of a small group of cells from the liquid medium in which they are dispersed. These cultures consist of cells in the rapidly dividing phase that are grown in a liquid nutrient media. In this type of culture, the first step involves the collection of the undifferentiated callus cells.

This mass arises from the proliferation of parent tissue, and consists of parenchymatous, amorphous and unorganised cells. Calluses are generally a result of injury at the incised ends of a stem or a root, but can initiate from any other parts such as the stem, root, leaf, flower or seed. The callus requires frequent sub-culturing for the following reasons:

- Exhaustion of nutrients over time
- Desiccation of agar
- Accumulation of cell metabolites, leading to toxicity effects on the culture.

One of the ways of avoiding this repeated sub-culturing is to freeze preserve the culture.

The callus when suspended in a liquid callus induction medium with all necessary nutrients and elements for optimal growth undergoes processes that convert all cells into undifferentiated cells. This cell suspension should be placed on a shaker to allow the dispersal of cell aggregates into smaller clumps and single cells, distributed uniformly throughout the liquid media. These cells will continuously grow until one of the factors gets depleted, leading to slowing and stoppage of cell growth. Prior to this final stage, cells are harvested and grown on a medium with specific proportions of growth hormones to activate growth of particular cells. For example, to induce formation of axillary and adventitious shoot, the medium should contain cytokinins. If auxins are present, it leads to the formation of adventitious roots. On complete development of plantlets, these are transplanted into the soil for further growth.

Isolation of single cells

Single cells can be isolated either from cultured tissues or from intact plant organs, the former being more convenient. An organized tissue (explant) is cultured into a callus (undifferentiated growth in solid form), which is later separated from the explant and transferred into fresh medium to get more tissue. When it is desired to obtain more tissue, pieces of undifferentiated calli are simply transferred to fresh medium and continuously agitated forming a suspension culture. Agitation of pieces is important to disperse them into smaller clumps and single cells. Besides, it helps to retain the cells uniformly distributed within the medium. It also promotes sufficient gaseous exchange.

It is possible to obtain suspension cultures with single cells starting from intact plant organs. This process involves grinding the tissue mechanically followed by cleaning, filtration and centrifugation. Alternatively, the excised plant parts can be treated with macero-enzymes to yield single cells.

Culture of single cells

Single cell cultures provide an opportunity to study properties and characteristics of plant cells and the factors that influence various physiological processes. These cultures are also useful in understanding cellular metabolic reactions.

Bergman's cell plating technique

Fresh cells are suspended in a liquid medium after filtering the cell aggregates. Culture medium with agar is cooled and maintained at 35°C in a water bath. Equal volumes of liquid and agar media are mixed and rapidly spread in a petridish. This helps in the even distribution of cells as a thin layer when the medium solidifies. The petri dishes are sealed with para film and examined with an inverted microscope. Single cells are marked on the outer surface of the dish. The plates are incubated in the dark at 25°C and cell colonies which develop from these marked single cells are used in the production of single-cell cultures.

Anther and pollen culture

When pollen grains are placed on suitable nutrient media like MS, a few form a callus although most of the others develop normally. Similarly, anthers can be cultured to yield embryos directly from pollen grains and further induced to develop true haploid plants. Provided there are explants and optimal nutrient condition for the donor plants, this method can yield hundreds of haploid plants originating from a single anther. For this type of culture to succeed, it is important that flower buds are excised during the first mitotic division in uni-nucleated microspore tetrads. It is possible to improve the chances of successful development of embryos by growing it on various nutrient media, and providing cold storage for a period ranging between a few days to several weeks.

Other methods such as filter paper raft-nurse technique and microchamber have also been developed to grow individual cells.

Suspension cultures

These can be maintained in either of the following two forms:

- ***Batch cultures***, which are initiated as single cells in 100–250 ml flasks. These can be further propagated by the regular transfer of small aliquots of suspension to a fresh medium.
- ***Continuous cultures*** that are maintained in a steady state for a long period. This involves draining out the used medium and adding fresh medium. During this process, if the cells separated from the drained medium are added back to the suspension culture, it is said to be *closed*. If a given volume of suspension culture is harvested and an equal volume of fresh culture is added, such cultures are called *open* continuous cultures. In open cultures, a steady state of suspension culture should be maintained for a long period.

Although continuous cultures have advantages, they require a lot of attention and it is difficult to procure the necessary equipment.

The medium used for suspension cultures is usually the same as for callus growth, except that agar is omitted. Slight changes in the auxin to cytokinin ratio may be necessary to allow appropriate dispersion of cells. Constant agitation of suspension cultures helps provide aeration and prevents clumping of cells.

Cell suspensions are often asynchronous as different cells exist at different stages of the cell cycle. Therefore, any of the following measures is essential to make them synchronous:

- ***Starvation*** Cells are starved of a nutrient that is necessary for cell division, such as a growth hormone. As a result, some of the cells are inhibited at the initial stages of growth. These arrested cells, when provided the requisite nutrient after some time, continue growing to obtain synchronous cell division.
- ***Inhibition*** Compounds such as thymidine, 5-aminouracil, and hydroxyurea that behave as DNA synthesis inhibitors can act by inhibiting the process of DNA synthesis, leading to cell arrest. A subsequent removal of inhibitors leads to the synchronous division of cells.

Clonal propagation or micropropagation

A wide variety of plant species can be conveniently propagated through cell, tissue or organ culture through clonal propagation or micropropagation. The major benefits of this technique are:

- Rapid multiplication of superior clones and maintenance of uniformity
- Multiplication of disease-free plants
- Multiplication of sexually derived sterile hybrids

Clonal propagation can be achieved by placing the sterilized shoot tips or axillary buds in a culture medium that has the capability of inducing multiple bud formation. This process passes through various stages such as:

Stage I Establishment of tissue in vitro

Stage II Multiplication of shoots (use a medium of the same composition as for the first stage)

Stage III Roots are formed and propagules are conditioned before they are transferred to the green house. At this stage, media composition will vary to allow root formation.

Stage IV Plantlets are grown in pots followed by field trials.

Bioreactors

Bioprocessors and bioreactors help to reduce the cost of plant tissue culture used in micropropagation and in the production of bio-active compounds. Using such technology, the production rate can be enhanced 10–1000 times. They are commonly found in biotechnology companies that are involved in large-scale production of biotechnology products.

Bioreactors use liquid culture media instead of a semi-solid agar medium. These are prepared and replaced regularly by using automatic devices that help to maintain consistent growth conditions. Bioreactors are used for organogenic or embryogenic tissue multiplication; they are later transferred to a bioprocessor and propagules of different sizes are separated from each other. Transferring these propagules into separate culture vessels allows them to grow and develop into plantlets, which are later transplanted, stored or shipped.

Synthetic seeds

These are somatic embryos encapsulated in a suitable matrix, such as, sodium alginate along with substances like mycorrhizae, insecticides, fungicides and herbicides. This technology helps to overcome problems in the storage and transportation of propagules for transplantation. They are also known as artificial seeds. The Bhabha Atomic Research Centre (BARC) has standardized and developed practices for preparing synthetic seeds of sandalwood and mulberry plants. Synthetic seeds have the following advantages:

- They do not show any loss of viability even when stored up to one year.
- They are easy to handle and transport.
- They can be directly sown in the soil like natural seeds and do not need hardening in the green house.

The major disadvantage of synthetic seeds is the high production cost.

This method has proved very successful in alfalfa and *Medicago sativa*. Artificial seeds of alfalfa can survive up to eight months when stored under dehydrated conditions. The alginate coating that is applied to these seeds does not appear to affect the seeds' transformation and germination rates.

Important applications of plant tissue culture

Plant tissue culture provides a variety of techniques for research in metabolic processes occurring in plant cells. However, it also has several commercial applications that make it easier and more convenient to produce phytoconsitutents that are useful for the pharmaceutical industry.

Some of the important applications of plant tissue culture are given below.

Production of useful phytoconstituents

- Various phytopharmaceuticals have been successfully isolated from plant tissue cultures. Examples include codeine, digoxin, morphine, nicotine, caffeine, diosgenin, vinblastine, atropine, quinine and quinidine.
- Large-scale production of biomass containing useful metabolites has been achieved. Examples include digitalis glycosides, steroidal hormone precursors derived from diosgenin, shikonin, opium alkaloids (codeine and morphine) and rosamarinic acid.
- Mass production of complex mixtures like rose and jasmine oil is possible.

- Some compounds which do not occur normally in a species can be found in the cell cultures of the species: for example,
    - o a new CNS active indole alkaloid, porcine, and a new anti-inflammatory agent, lignin;
    - o unusual ether lipids have been isolated from algae cultures of *Chlorella fusca*.
- The rate of production of secondary metabolites from tissue culture technology has been shown to be remarkably higher than from the intact plant. For example, shikonin from Lithospermum, berberine from Coptis, jatrorrhizini from Berberis, rosamarinic acid from Coleus. The yield is also higher.

In recent years, there is an increasing use of plant cell suspension cultures and immobilized cells for the commercial scale production of chemicals, because this method provides various advantages in comparison with the process of extraction from whole plants.

- Tissue cultures are not influenced by the vagaries of environmental conditions since they are maintained under controlled conditions. Therefore, high quality is consistently achieved in cell cultures.
- The production schedule can be estimated and controlled in the laboratory or industry.

Secondary metabolites

The term secondary metabolites refers to certain organic compounds which are not directly required or involved in the growth, development or reproduction of organisms. A deficiency of these secondary metabolites will not cause death of the plant. In some species it may have no effect at all, and in others, it can lead to long-term damage in the characteristic properties of the plants. Many of these compounds are synthesized only at particular periods during the developmental stages, but not during the rest of the lifetime of the plant. Various secondary metabolites have been discovered as having useful properties and since ancient times, these have been used in traditional medicine as curatives and food additives. Common examples of secondary metabolites include steroids, terpenoids, alkaloids, glycosides, essential oils and pigments. Tables 12.3 and 12.4 list some important secondary metabolites derived from plants by using tissue culture techniques.

Table 12.3 Types of secondary metabolites

Small secondary metabolites	
Alkaloids	Hyoscyamine, atropine, cocaine, codeine, morphine, vincristine, vinblastine
Glycosides	Glucosinolates, nojirimycin
	Azadirachtin, artemisinin, steroid, tetrahydrocannabinol
Saponins	Plant steroids
Phenols	Reservaratrol
Big secondary metabolites	
Polyketides	Erythromycin
Non-ribosomal peptides	Vancomycin, gramicidin, bacitracin

Table 12.4 Secondary metabolites obtained by tissue culture

Plant species	Secondary metabolites
Catharanthus roseus	Vincristine, ajmalicine, ajmalthine, serpentine
Cinchona officinalis	Quinine
Digitalis lanata	Digoxin, reserpine
Papaver somniferum	Morphine
Glycyrrhiza glabra	Glycyrrhizin

The quantities of these chemicals produced in cell culture are considerably lower than in whole plants. However, by manipulating certain physiological and biochemical conditions, it is possible to substantially increase their levels. In certain cases, cell cultures can produce about two to ten times more of these secondary metabolites than the mother plants.

Table 12.5 Comparison of yield of various secondary metabolites from mother plants and cell culture

Compound	Plant species	Yields (% dry weight)	
		Culture	Plant
Shikonin	*Lithospermum erythrorhizon*	20	1.5
Ginsenside	*Panax ginseng*	27	4.5
Ajmalicine	*Catharanthus roseus*	1.0	1.5
Berberine	*Thallictrum minor*	10	0.01
Nicotine	*Nicotiana tabacum*	3.4	2.0
Diosgenin	*Dioscorea deltoidea*	2	2

Biochemical conversions

Various reactions that are chemically difficult even in the presence of enzymes or microorganisms, have been shown to occur with ease in plant cell cultures. The common biotransformation reactions include methylation, demethylation, acetylation, reduction, glycosylation and hydroxylation. These biotransformation reactions using plant cell strains play a significant role in the production of compounds that possess medicinal value. One of the areas of interest over the past few years where such reactions have been widely studied is the biotransformation of steroids using microbial and plant cell cultures. The best example of such reactions is the biotransformation of digitoxin to cardiac glycosides using low-cost precursor substances as a substrate to yield highly valuable and expensive products. Some examples include:

- A suspension culture of *Digitalis lanata* can convert digitoxin or methyl digitoxin into digoxin or methyl digoxin, which have great medicinal value in the treatment of heart diseases. The conversion rate for this transformation has been estimated to be as high as 15% in 24 hours and 70% in 7 days.
- Datura cell cultures have shown a potential to convert hydroquinone to arbutin, a diuretic and urinary antiseptic, by the process of glycosylation.
- Cell cultures of *Stevia rebaudiana* and *Digitalis purpurea* can convert steviol into steviobiocide and stevioside, which are compounds with sweetness about 100 times greater than that of cane sugar.

Plant improvement

Tissue culture techniques are of great importance to the improvement of various aspects of plants. Some of the uses are mentioned below:

- In vitro production and propagation of virus-free material. This is especially true with old clones and material propagated through the use of vegetative techniques. Tissue culture techniques make it easier to carry out in vitro fertilization, because they help to overcome self-incompatibility and cause ploidy changes.
- Screening studies at the tissue or cellular level to find out resistance to disease, toxins and stress conditions can be carried out.
- Induction and selection of mutants, especially in connection with selection of crops. Using various mutagenic treatments, it is possible to increase the frequency of mutations several fold. This, in turn makes screening of millions of cells possible. Selection of cells is done by adding the toxic substance against which resistance is sought in the mutant cells and choosing the type which shows the desired resistance. This strategy has been used to develop and isolate cell lines that are resistant to amino acid analogues, antibiotics, herbicides and fungal toxins.

Production of single cell proteins

The term single cell proteins (SCP) was coined in 1966, and is defined as any microbial biomass from both unicellular and multicellular bacteria, yeasts, filamentous fungi and algae which can be used as food or feed additives. Generally, the microbial biomass contains around 45%–55% proteins, although a few species of bacteria exhibit a protein content that is as high as 80%.

Elucidation of biogenetic pathways

Cell cultures have also been used to help elucidate the individual steps in biosynthetic pathways of various alkaloids. For example,

- cultured cells of the solanaceous plant *Anisodus acutangulus* have been used to study the conversion of plant hyoscyamine to hyoscine;
- various cell cultures of *Papaver somniferum* have been used to study the biosynthetic pathway of benzyl isoquinoline alkaloids, particularly morphine and codeine.

Limitations of tissue culture

- There is still only incomplete information available about the exact process that takes place during de-differentiation in the callus. Similarly, there is insufficient knowledge of the process of inducing shoot bud initiation.
- Many cultures although useful for various applications, have been found to suffer from a lack of sufficient stability.
- In many cases, there are no effective methods for identification of variants.
- Knowledge of important physiological and biochemical processes in plants and information of the molecular and cellular mechanisms that regulate important agronomical traits in plants is still limited.
- Plant cells behave differently from microorganisms in cultures. Bacterial cells separate when they divide forming equivalent individuals. In plant cells, the daughter cells remain attached to form a mass of cells. This mass is exposed to differing environments on its outer and inner surface. Due to this, the cells present in the inner regions of the mass do not have the same access to the nutrients present in the culture medium. This leads to significant biogenetic difference in the same culture.
- Although this technique has been tried with many crops or medicinal plants, not all of them show an ability to regenerate different varieties from cultured cells. In this sense, it is said that plant regeneration is more of an art than a science.
- The application of plant tissue culture to crop improvement is still limited in its reach because identification of traits is possible only in the case of ones that have an expression at the cellular level. For example, it may be possible to identify the genes for traits such as tolerance to heavy metals, salts or herbicides. However, a similar identification is not possible presently for various other traits such as flowering time or high yield, which are under the control of a different set of genes.

12.3 PLANT CELL CULTURE AND SECONDARY METABOLITES

Production of shikonin by tissue culture

This is one of the best examples of the commercial success of tissue culture. Shikonin is a red naphthoquinone, found naturally in the roots of various Boraginaceae species, such as *Lithospermum erythrorhizon*. The dried root of the plant, called zicao, is a useful herb in Chinese medicine. Shikonin contains various biologically active components, with the major one being zicao, that has anti-tumour action. It helps in quicker healing of wounds and inhibits action of HIV. Shikonin has also been used as a textile dye, food colourant and cosmetic due to its bright red colour. Shikonin is the first plant secondary metabolite to be commercially produced by plant cell culture.

This method of production was developed by Tabata and Fujita of Kyoto University, Japan in 1985. They observed that cultures of *L. erythrorhizon* could produce shikonin. They also noticed that production of this pigment could be increased by selecting cells showing high productivity. After extensive investigation of the factors regulating metabolism, such as effects of temperature, light, wavelength, growth hormones and carbon and nitrogen sources on production of shikonin, they came up with a two-stage culture system:

1. In the first stage, the cells are grown with agar.
2. In the next stage, the cells are transferred to an agar-free medium with high calcium that helps to increase the final yield of shikonin.

According to Tabata and Fujita,

- The cell culture procedure for making shikonin is about 800 times more productive than the traditional plant cultivation method.
- Shikonin content of the cultured cells is about 15 times higher than in the plant material.
- It takes less than a month for producing shikonin by this method compared to the 48 months required for actual cultivation.
- Production of shikonin by plant cell culture is more economical when compared to the production by chemical synthesis.

COMMERCIAL PRODUCTION OF SHIKONIN

High-yielding clone cells are used as the inoculum and are maintained in jar fermenters. The inoculum is first added to a 200-litre fermenter (first stage) containing the MG-5 medium for culture growth. After nine days, the cells are filtered and inoculated into a 750-litre fermenter (second stage) containing M-9 shikonin production medium and incubated for 14 days.

The cells are harvested by simple filtration, extracted with *n*-hexane followed by hydrolysis with 2% pottassium hydroxide and recrystallisation to give pure shikonin. A 750-litre bioreactor containing 600 litres of medium were found to yield 1.2 kg of shikonin in two weeks. This was in sharp contrast to 9 kg of shikonin obtained from Lithospermum roots cultivated on one hectare after about four years.

Factors influencing shikonin production

- Temperature range of 20–25°C is most favourable.
- No specific light is required.
- Natural auxins such as IAA (indole acetic acid) enhance, whereas synthetic auxins such as naphthalene acetic acid inhibit shikonin production.
- The nutrients required are:
  - Sucrose is the best source of carbon whereas other sugars inhibit oduction.
  - Total nitrogen content should be maintained constant since a decrease has a negative impact on shikonin production.
  - Trace nutrients such as copper, calcium, iron, boron and sulphur tend to increase shikonin production.
  - Agar in combination with the Linsmaier–Skoog medium is used to prepare culture media.
- Dissolved oxygen in the medium must be at a concentration of 6–6.4 ppm.

12.4 BIOTRANSFORMATION

Biotransformation is defined as the process in which the functional groups of organic compounds are modified by living cells. This was initially investigated for applications in microbiology. Presently, biotransformation is being studied with respect to plant cell cultures for producing secondary metabolites.

Plant cell cultures are less capable of biotransformation reactions as compared to microbial catalytic systems because of slower growth curve and difficulty in maintaining sterility of the culture.

The basic step in plant cell culture biotransformation reactions is performed using cell suspension cultures with the compound to be transformed. This leads to a reaction that yields the product which is later harvested from the culture. In some instances, cells with the potential to aid a biotransformation reaction are immobilized within a matrix and are allowed to come into contact with immobilized enzymes, leading to the formation of secondary metabolites.

Prerequisites for biotransformation through cell culture

Biotransformation potential

The basic requirement for carrying out such reactions is the biotransformation potential within the substrate. This substrate should be capable of easy assimilation by the cells within the culture and it should be able to reach the appropriate location without any degradation. More importantly, this substrate should not cause any toxicity to the cell culture and once the product begins to form, the rate of its formation should be far greater than the rate of its catabolism.

Selection of the right growth regulator

This is of importance, because these substances exert a significant influence on the process of differentiation or de-differentiation of a culture. This in turn has an effect on the synthesis of certain enzymes, and can therefore affect the formation of secondary metabolites.

It is preferable to use enzymes that are functional group-specific; examples include enzymes such as glycosidases, peroxidases and dehydrogenases. These are more flexible in their action as compared to substrate-specific enzymes which act on only certain substrates.

A few common reaction types and chemical groups involved in biotransformation by cell culture are shown below.

Reduction

$C{=}C \rightarrow CH_2{-}CH_2$

$C{=}C \rightarrow -CO- \rightarrow -CH_2{-}CH_2{-}CO- \rightarrow CH_2CH_2CHOH$

$CO \rightarrow CHOH$

$CHO \rightarrow CH_2OH \rightarrow CH_3$

Oxidation

$CH_3 \rightarrow CH_2OH$

$CH_3 \rightarrow COOH$

$CH_2OH \rightarrow CHO$

$CHOH \rightarrow CO$

$CH_2{-}CH_2 \rightarrow CH{=}CH$

$CH_2{-}CH_2{-}NH_2 \rightarrow CH_2COOH$

$=S \rightarrow S{=}O$

Hydroxylation

CH → C–OH

CH_2 → CH–OH

NH_2 → NH–OH

Epoxidation

CH=CH → 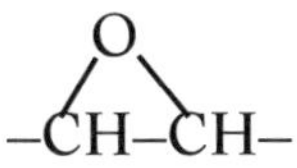

Glycoxylation

OH → O-glucose

OH → O-rhamnose

OH → O-apiose

COOH → COO-glucose

CH → C-glucose

N → ≡ N^+-arabinose

Esterification

OH→ O-Ac

OH→ $O-COCH_2N(Et)_2$

OH → O-palmitate

OH → O-malonate

OH → O-succinate

COOH → COO-malate

Methylation

OH → $O-CH_3$

≡ N → ≡ N^+-CH_3

≡ N^+– CH → =NH

Isomerization

Trans ↔ cis

D form → L form

β-OH → α-OH

Enhancement of product yield

Biotransformation reactions involving plant cell cultures take longer when compared to microbial cultures, because the former have slower rates of growth and metabolism. There is a significant difference in the potential for production of secondary metabolites between cultures of different species of a plant and sometimes within the same cultivar. The best way to improve the yield from such cultures is to select cell strains that possess a high potential for the desired biotransformation reactions.

Selecting high-yielding plants to initiate cell cultures is a valuable method of increasing yields. For example, it is found that using *Catharanthus roseus* plants with high yields of alkaloids gives suspension cultures that also give higher yields of alkaloid. However, this does not always hold true as is seen in the case of *Digitalis lanata*. When high-digoxin yielding *Digitalis lanata* was used to initiate cultures, it was found that the culture had completely lost its capacity to biotransform digitoxin to digoxin.

Productivity of cell cultures can be enhanced by exact control of various influencing factors such as temperature, light, rate of agitation, composition of the nutrient medium and proportion of growth regulators.

Secondary compounds produced by biotransformation

Cardiac glycosides

Using digitoxin—a secondary glycoside of *Digitalis purpurea*—as a substrate in cell cultures of *Digitalis lanata* it has been possible to produce digoxin, which is a more effective cardiotonic.

Cell cultures of *Digitalis lanata* have also shown a capacity to bring about the successful biotransformation of β-methyl digitoxin to β-methyl digoxin(Fig. 12.6).

Steroids

Sterols such as sitosterol, which are found in higher plants and animal sterols such as cholesterol, have been transformed to diosgenin using plant cell cultures of *Dioscorea deltoidea*. Diosgenin serves as an important precursor for the synthesis of various steroidal hormones that have medicinal significance (Figs 12.7 and 12.8).

Terpenoids

These are intermediates produced along the acetate–mevalonate pathway. Monoterpenoids are important components of essential oils and are widely used in food flavouring, perfumes and pharmaceutical industries. It has been found that cell cultures of *Lavendula angustifolia*, which are devoid of monoterpenoids, have the capability to transform added aldehydes such as geranial, citronellal and perillaldehyde to their corresponding alcohols (Fig. 12.9).

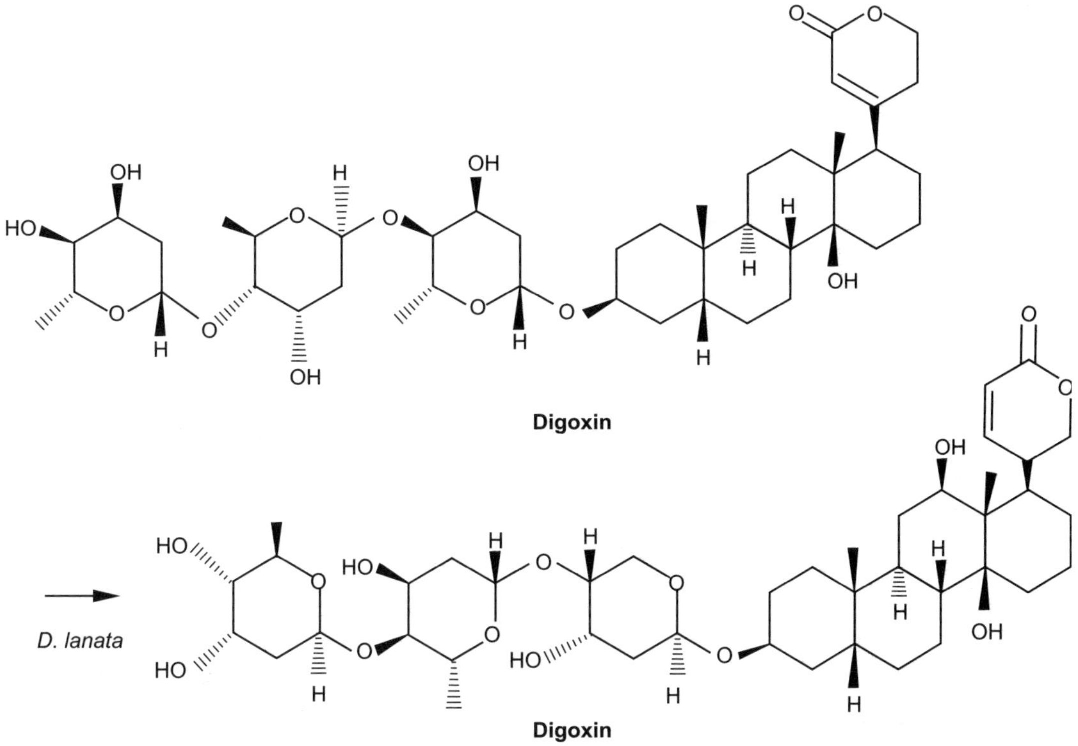

Fig. 12.6 Biotransformation of digitoxin to digoxin

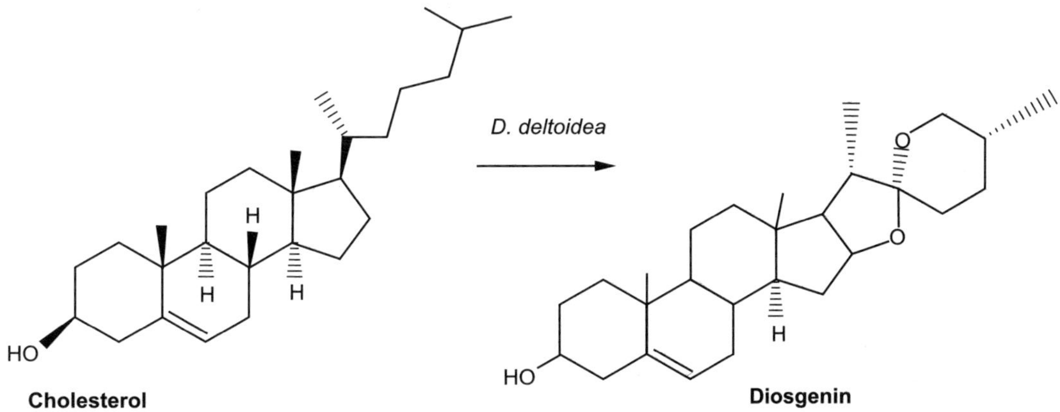

Fig. 12.7 Biotransformation of cholesterol to diosgenin

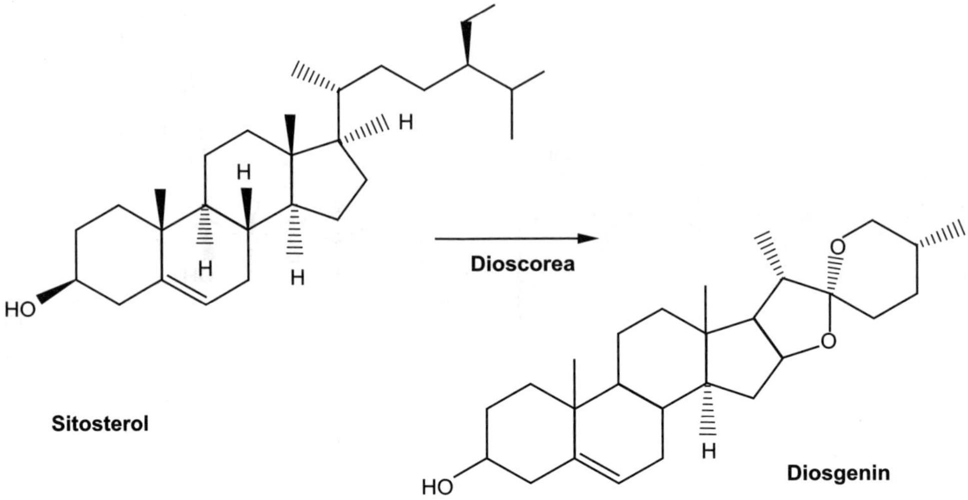

Fig. 12.8 Biotransformation of sitosterol to diosgenin

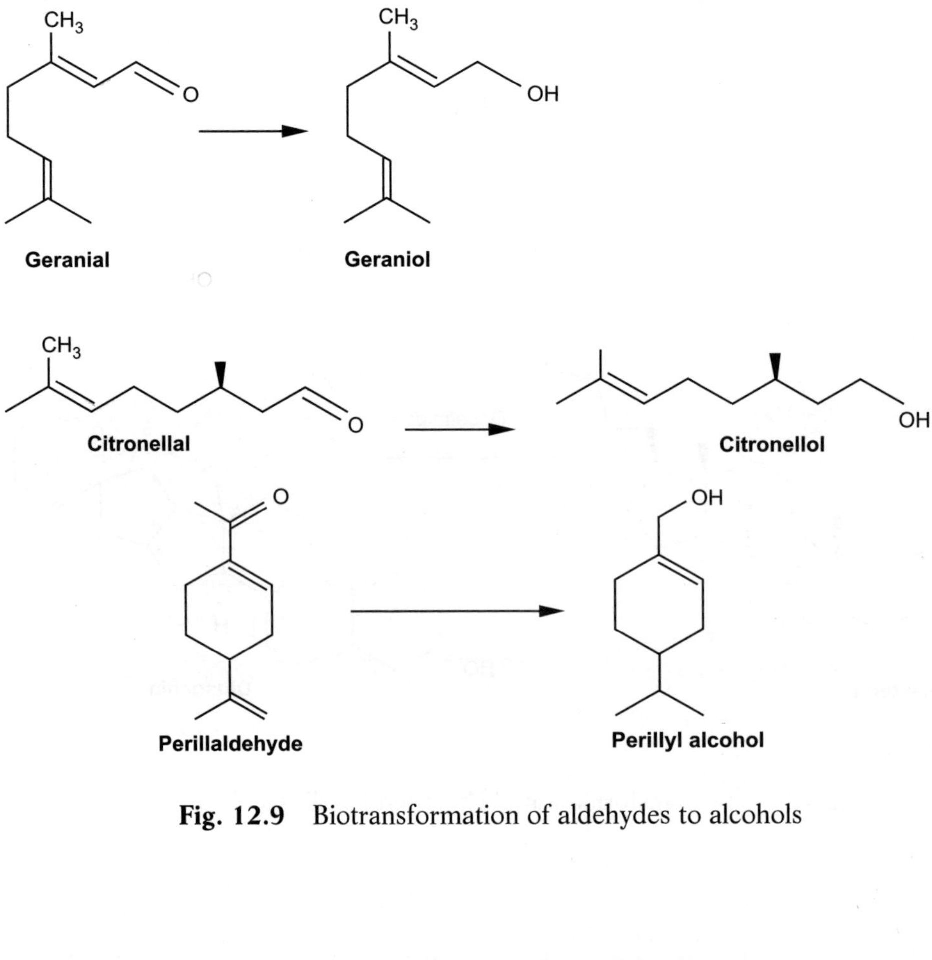

Fig. 12.9 Biotransformation of aldehydes to alcohols

Similarly, cell cultures of different Mentha species have been shown to transform (–) Menthone to (+) Neomenthol by the reduction of C=O group to –OH group. Similarly, (+) Pulegone has been biotransformed to (+) Isomenthone through the reduction of the double bond (Fig. 12.10).

Other interesting examples include:

- Diterepenoid biotransformation using a cell suspension of *Stevia reboudiana* and *D. purpurea*, in which glycosidation of sSteviol occurs to yield stevioside (a sweet glycoside which is 300 times sweeter than sugar).
- Hydroxylation of Coumarin at position 7 to yield umbelliferone, using cell cultures of *Catharanthus roseus* and *Conium maculatum*.
- Cultures of *Lithospermum erythrorhizon*, *Gardenia jasnoids* and *Nicotiana tabacum* show an ability to transform the aglycone esculetin to a glucoside esculin (Fig. 12.11).
- There are also reports of simple phenolic substrates like salicylaldehyde (Fig. 12.12) and salicyl alcohol (Fig. 12.13) being glycosylated to isosalicin rather than to the glucoside salicin when placed in cell suspension cultures of *Datura inoxia*. This same culture has also shown an ability to convert hydroquinone and vanillin to their respective glycosides arbutin and glucovanillin.

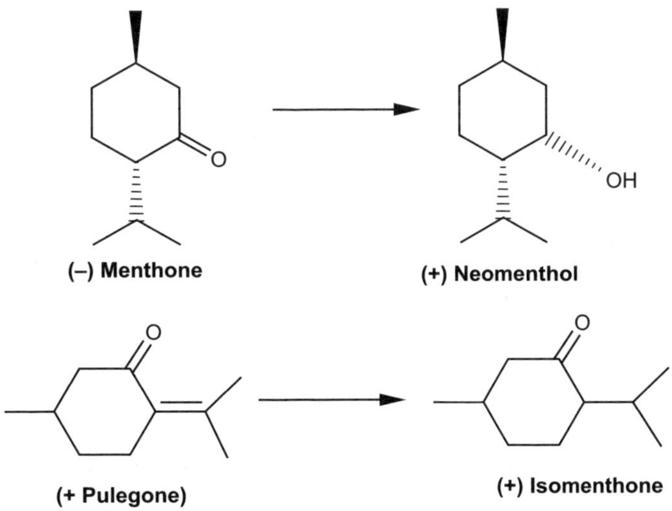

Fig. 12.10 Biotransformation of menthone to menthol

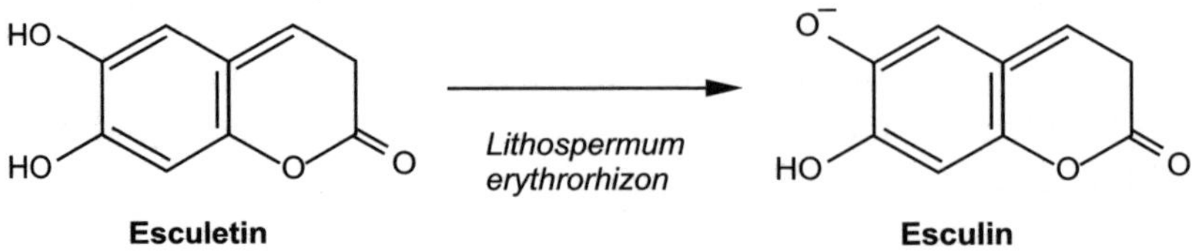

Fig. 12.11 Transformation of esculetin to esculin

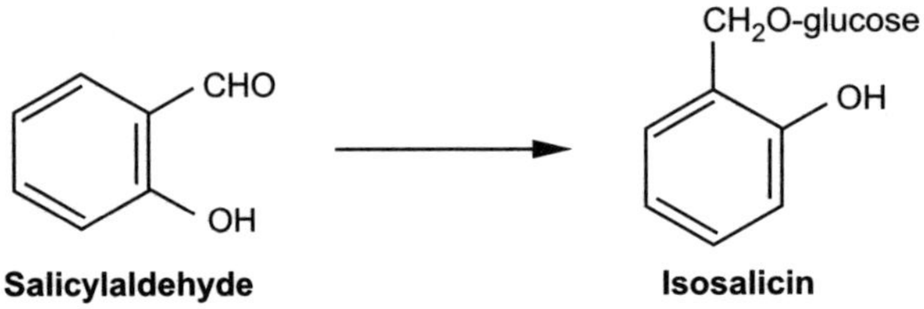

Fig. 12.12 Glycosylation of salicylaldehyde

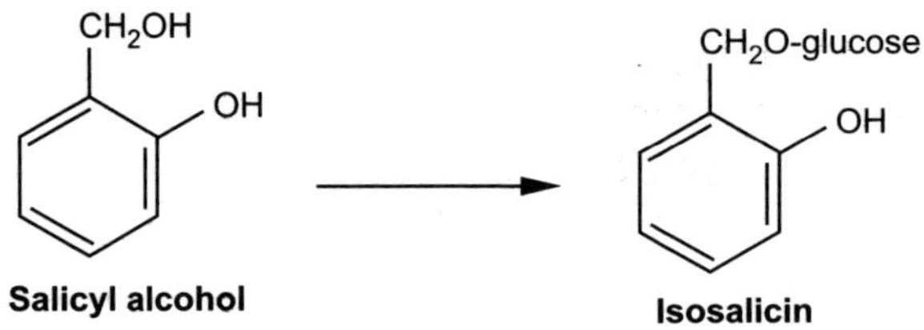

Fig. 12.13 Glycosylation of salicyl alcohol

SUMMARY

- Plant tissue culture is used for propagating plants under sterile conditions, often resulting in the production of clones. Plant tissue culture relies on the property of totipotency of plant cells.
- Various factors that enable the success of tissue culture include a suitable nutrient medium, presence of growth regulators and the maintenance of required conditions of temperature, pH and humidity.
- The rate of production of secondary metabolites from tissue culture technology is remarkably higher than from the intact plant.
- Plant tissue cultures show the ability for various reactions like methylation, demethylation, acetylation, reduction, glycosylation and hydroxylation.These biotransformations have been used in the production of various phytochemicals.

Exercises

Long answers

1. Define tissue culture and discuss its applications.
2. Discuss in vitro production of secondary metabolites.
3. Outline the techniques and methods of single cell culture.
4. Discuss in brief the requirements of tissue culture.
5. Describe the factors that affect plant tissue culture.

Short answers

6. Write a short note on the production of shikonin.
7. Discuss the role of growth hormones in plants.
8. Explain biotransformation using tissue culture technology.
9. Describe the types of reactions that occur during plant tissue culture.

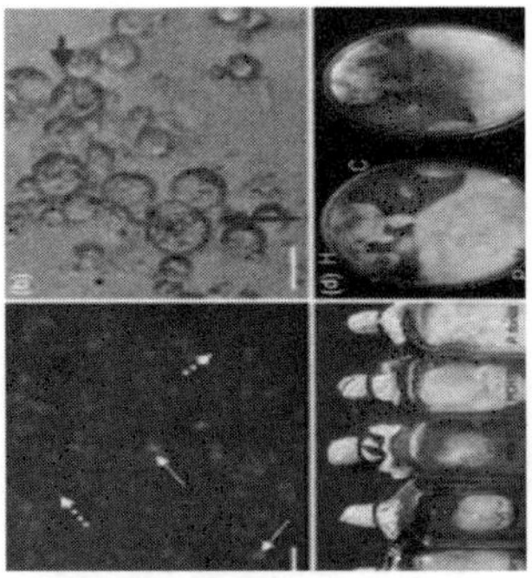

13

Protoplast Technology

In This Chapter, You Will Learn

- The definition and uses of protoplasts
- The different methods of protoplast isolation and purification
- What is protoplast fusion technology
- Somatic hybridization and its applications
- What are transgenic plants
- The methods of genetic transformation of plants
- Plant cell immobilization

13.1 PROTOPLASTS

The cell wall in plants plays an important role in processes connected with structure and function. However, it serves as a barrier and prevents the direct transfer of DNA. This does not allow cell fusion that is essential for the production of hybrid seeds. It has been observed that removal of the cell wall does not cause any significant loss of viability. Those plant cells from which the cell wall has been removed are called protoplasts. In other words, a protoplast is defined as 'a plant, bacterial or fungal cell that has its cell wall completely or partially removed using either mechanical or enzymatic means'. These protoplasts are unique in plant cell culture as they exist as separate cells, and do not share any cytoplasmic continuity with the neighbouring cells.

Cell walls are made of different polysaccharides. Production of protoplasts, therefore, depends on the process of digesting cell walls with a mixture of the appropriate enzymes that degrade polysaccharides. Table 13.1 lists the common enzymes used in plant cells to remove the cell wall.

Table 13.1 Enzymes used to remove polysaccharides in the cell wall

Type of cell	Enzyme
Plant cells	Cellulase, pectinase, xylanase
Gram-positive bacteria	Lysozyme (+EDTA)
Fungal cells	Chitinase

Cellulase enzymes are used to digest cellulose in plant cell walls. Pectinase enzymes break down the pectin that binds cells together. The protoplast produced by removal of the cell wall is spherical. The process of digestion requires prior incubation of cells in an osmoticum, which renders the cell walls susceptible to digestion. An *osmoticum* is a solution which has higher concentration than the contents of the cells that it holds. As a result, this solution causes the cells to plasmolyze. Debris generated by this process requires filtration or centrifugation to be separated from the suspension. At the end of this, the suspension is again centrifuged to give the final protoplasts in the form of a pellet. The entire process of digestion, centrifuging and storage should be carried out using an isotonic solution. This is important to avoid rupturing the plasma membrane, because the protoplast without the cell wall is highly sensitive to osmotic stress.

13.2 ISOLATION OF PROTOPLASTS

Protoplasts can be produced by two methods:

- *Mechanical method* Here, cells are kept in a suitable plasmolyticum (in plasmolysed cells, the protoplasts have shrunk away from the cell wall) and subsequently cut with a fine knife.
- *Enzymatic method* This method consists of digesting the cell wall using hydrolytic enzymes.

Mechanical method

Here, cells are kept in a suitable plasmolyticum —the protoplasts that have shrunk away from the cell wall in the plasmolyzed cells— and subsequently cut with a fine knife. This causes the release of protoplasts from the cells which have been cut through the cell wall. When this tissue is de-plasmolyzed, the protoplasts move out. This method is best suited for separating protoplasts present in vacuolated cells such as those seen in onion bulbs, scales and radish. However, this method does not work with protoplasts present in meristematic and non-vacuolated cells. Therefore, it has limited application.

Enzymatic method

This is the most widely used method to isolate protoplasts, because large quantities of intact protoplasts can be produced with minimal osmotic shrinkage. In a few instances, it may be necessary to use a combination of mechanical and enzymatic methods. In such cases, cells are first separated mechanically, followed by enzymatic treatment to isolate the protoplasts.

This method is useful in isolating protoplasts from a variety of tissues such as roots, leaves, pollen, in vitro shoot cultures, callus and cell suspensions.

Leaves are the most commonly used part for protoplast isolation using the following steps:

1. The fully expanded leaves of a 10-week old plant are sterilized by dipping into 70% ethanol for about 1 minute. They are then treated with 2% solution of sodium hypochlorite for 20–30 minutes, and rinsed three times with sterile distilled water. All subsequent operations are carried out under the laminar air flow unit.
2. The lower epidermis of sterilized leaves is carefully peeled off and the leaves are cut into small pieces, after which, the protoplasts can be isolated either by the direct or the sequential method. In the direct or one-step method, there is simultaneous treatment with both macero-enzyme (or pectinase) and cellulase. In the sequential or two-step method, cells are treated first using macero-enzyme and then with cellulase to isolate the protoplasts. It has been found that the yield of protoplasts is higher in the one-step method, but the protoplasts from the sequential method are better for culture studies.

Direct method

The leaf segments are incubated overnight with an enzyme mixture at 25°C for 15–18 hours. Later, this mixture is teased gently to free the protoplasts. The mixture is then filtered through fine wire gauze to remove leaf debris and centrifuged at 100 g for 1 minute. This procedure is repeated three times to ensure that the protoplasts form a pellet. The supernatant is removed, and the protoplasts are washed using in succession, a 13% sorbitol solution and a 20% sucrose solution. This suspension is then centrifuged at a speed of 200 g for 1 minute. The cleaned protoplasts float up and the debris which settles down can be removed easily.

Sequential method

The leaf segments are treated with mixture A (0.5% macero-enzyme and 0.3% K-dextran sulphate in 13% mannitol at pH 5.8). This is subjected to vacuum infiltration for 5 minutes, and then transferred to a water bath maintained at 25°C. After low agitation for 15 minutes, the enzyme mixture is replenished with fresh enzyme mixture A and the leaf segments are incubated for another hour. The mixture so obtained is subjected to filtration through nylon mesh, and centrifuged at 100 g for 1 minute, then washed thrice with 13% mannitol to yield a pure sample of isolated cells. This is followed by an incubation of these cells with enzyme mixture B (2% cellulose in 13% solution of mannitol at pH 5.4) for more than 90 minutes at 30°C. Centrifuging this mixture at 100 g for 1 minute causes the protoplasts to form a pellet that can be subsequently cleaned three times as in the direct method.

13.3 PURIFICATION OF ISOLATED PROTOPLASTS

The isolated protoplasts are often contaminated with cell debris and broken cell organelles. Purification by separating these contaminants can be done using two common methods.

SEDIMENTATION AND WASHING

Centrifuging the crude protoplast suspension at low speed (50–100 g) for 5 minutes causes the intact protoplasts to form a pellet. The supernatant which contains the cell debris can then be removed by using a pipette. Re-suspending the pellet in fresh culture media that contains mannitol and re-washing it yields a clean, pure protoplast preparation.

FLOTATION

Since the protoplasts have a lower density in comparison to other cell debris, it is possible to use osmotic gradients which cause the protoplasts to float as cell debris sediments. A concentrated solution of mannitol, sorbitol and sucrose can be used as a gradient at an appropriate speed. Protoplasts collect at the top of the tube following centrifugation and can be removed with a pipette. This method is preferable because it is less damaging to the protoplast.

13.4 PROTOPLAST VIABILITY

The viability of the protoplasts produced can be tested by the following methods:

- Testing for the presence of cytoplasmic streaming
- Exclusion of Evans blue dye
- Change in protoplast size due to a change in the level of osmoticum (a solution causing change in osmotic pressure)
- Presence of photosynthetic and respiratory activity

Currently, the most common method uses dyes like fluorescein diacetate (FDA), phenosafranin and calcofluor white (CFW). As FDA accumulates inside the plasma membrane, viable protoplasts show green or white fluorescence. They should be examined within 5–15 minutes of the treatment because FDA dissociates after this period. A 0.1% solution of phenosafranin can detect dead protoplasts which turn red in its presence. Viable protoplasts, however, remain unstained even after immersion for 2 hours in the stain solution. CFW (0.1% v/v) can detect re-formation of cell wall in viable protoplasts. This regeneration of the cell wall appears as a ring of fluorescence.

The number of protoplasts present in a suspension can be counted using a modified Rosenthal haemocytometer. The protoplast suspended in a known volume (10 ml) of washing solution is introduced beneath the cover slip. The number of protoplasts enclosed by the triple-lined square is counted (*n*) including those touching the top and left edges but not the bottom or right edges. The number is calculated per millilitre. The total yield for a volume of 10 ml is usually $5n \times 104$.

13.5 PROTOPLAST CULTURE

Culturing of protoplasts can be done either within a thin layer of liquid medium that has been embedded in agarose, or inside a totally liquid medium. It can also be done on the surface of a solid medium or inside droplets of agarose that are suspended in liquid. The exact method of culturing used depends on the particular species being studied. Generally, the use of a liquid medium is preferred because it is easier to adjust the cell density and osmotic pressure.

A medium similar to that used for cell suspension cultures is used, with a few modifications to induce sustained division of protoplasts.

- Ammonium ions are reduced or removed from the media because they are known to be detrimental to protoplast survival.
- Sugar and sugar alcohols such as mannitol and sorbitol are added to adjust the osmotic pressure of the enzyme mixtures, protoplast washing solutions and culture media.
- Sucrose is used as the carbon source because the tissues derived from protoplasts are known to be non-photosynthetic.
- Whichever culturing method is used, the protoplasts start developing cell walls within 2–4 days. This can be detected by staining with 0.1% CFW. The first division occurs within 2–7 days. The next step is the formation of multicellular colonies after 2–3 weeks. By another 2 weeks, these colonies can be used for regeneration of plants.

The first step in the regeneration consists of transferring the callus to a medium that can initiate differentiation. This callus shows properties similar to those of the callus obtained from cells. The calli further differentiate into shoots; root formation is also possibile. After this stage, the plantlets can be transferred to pots. Plants regenerated from protoplasts show greater variation than those regenerated from a meristem, a stem segment or a leaf disc.

Sub-protoplasts

These are protoplasts that do not have all the contents of plant cells. They can be of the following types:

Cytoplasts They have no nucleus but contain the entire cytoplasm of a cell or a part of the cell and may sometimes also lead to the transfer of a part of the genome. They are often used for somatic hybridization.

Karyoplasts or ***miniprotoplasts*** They contain a nucleus surrounded by some cytoplasm and the original outer plasma membrane.

Microprotoplasts They contain only a few chromosomes and a fraction of the cytoplasm.

Microplasts They contain only a fraction of the cytoplasm and the outer membrane.

13.6 USES OF PROTOPLASTS

- The main use of protoplasts is in the study of membrane biology, which includes the uptake of viruses and macromolecules.
- Protoplasts find wide application in DNA transformation during the creation of genetically modified organisms, where there is a need to remove the cell wall that otherwise blocks DNA from entering the cell.
- Protoplasts can be used for the regeneration of whole plants by first converting them into plant cells that develop into a callus. This callus then develops shoots through plant tissue culture. The tissue culture medium should contain the correct balance of plant growth regulators.
- Protoplast fusion is one of the methods of plant breeding that involves the fusion of plants from distantly related or unrelated species, which cannot otherwise reproduce sexually, due to genetic incompatibility. Such fusion leads to the formation of plants that combine the desirable characteristics of both species like disease resistance and cold tolerance.

Protoplast fusion

Fusion of protoplasts can be achieved through the use of chemical or electrical techniques that cause a temporary destabilization of the plasma membranes. This leads to the formation of pores that form a cytoplasmic linkage between adjacent protoplasts.

Spontaneous fusion
When the cell walls are enzymatically degraded during the process of isolation, a few protoplasts in close proximity might fuse. The resulting entities are called homokaryons

or homokaryocytes, and each one contains anywhere between 2 and 40 nuclei. It is also possible to induce such spontaneous fusion by bringing the protoplasts into close contact with each other using micromanipulators or micropipettes. This type of fusion is more likely in protoplasts obtained from young leaves.

Induced fusion

Fusion can be induced between protoplasts from two different species, called as *inter-specific fusion,* or between protoplasts from two different sources for the same species. This type of fusion is useful for somatic hybridization. The agent used to induce fusion is called a fusogen and can be a chemical compound or an electric current. The fusogen draws the protoplasts together, thereby causing them to adhere to one another, leading to fusion.

Chemical fusion

Many aqueous solutions of salts such as sodium and potassium chloride, and sodium and potassium nitrate have been found useful in inducing chemical fusion of plant protoplasts. Other chemicals such as dextran sulphate, polyvinyl alcohol, lysolecithin and polyethylene glycol (PEG) have also been used.

Treatment with sodium nitrate

This method has shown success with protoplasts from root tips of oat and maize seedlings. However, it is not very useful with protoplasts that are highly vacuolated because it shows a low fusion frequency. In this method, the isolated protoplasts are suspended in a mixture (5% sodium nitrate in 10% sucrose solution) that induces fusion. When this suspension is incubated on a water bath maintained at a temperature of 35°C, it causes fusion. The mixture can be centrifuged, followed by re-suspending the pellet and incubated for more cycles. The mixture is finally replaced by a liquid medium and the protoplasts in this mixture are incubated again. This procedure is repeated one or two times and then the protoplasts are plated on a solid medium. The fusion of protoplasts can be confirmed throughout the process by examining under an inverted microscope.

Treatment with calcium ions at high pH

In this method, the protoplasts are placed in a solution that induces fusion and then centrifuged for half an hour at 50 g. Following this, the tubes are incubated in a water bath for 45 minutes at a temperature of 37°C. A 0.05M solution of calcium chloride in 0.4M mannitol is used and the pH of this solution is adjusted to 10.5. This method causes about 20%–50% of the protoplasts to fuse, and yields good results in some cases, but is often toxic because of the high pH.

Polyethylene glycol (PEG) treatment

This gives consistently high frequency of fusion, and also has low cytotoxic potential as compared to other methods. It is one of the methods generally used for fusing protoplasts obtained from unrelated plant taxa. Protoplasts can be treated with PEG in two ways to cause agglutination.

1. Provided there are a sufficient number of protoplasts available, 1 ml of culture medium containing the suspended protoplasts is added to 1 ml of a 56% solution of PEG. This tube is shaken for 5 seconds, and the protoplasts are allowed to sediment for 10 min, followed by a wash using the growth medium. The suspension is then examined to check if fusion has occurred successfully.
2. When protoplasts are available only in very little quantity, it is preferable to use drop cultures. Here, the two protoplasts to be fused are mixed in equal quantities. About 4–6 microdrops (100 μl each) are placed in a small petri plate at room temperature for 5–10 minutes. After this, 2–3 microdrops (50 μ each) of PEG are added along the sides of each petri plate, and the plate is then incubated for 30 min at a temperature of 24°C to cause the protoplasts to agglutinate. Placing a cover glass in the centre of the petri plate prior to pouring the protoplast suspension prevents the protoplasts from sticking to the floor of the petri plate. Besides, it also makes handling, fixing, staining and examination of the protoplasts more convenient.

   Following the PEG treatment, protoplasts are carefully washed to achieve complete fusion. The fused protoplasts are then placed in the culture medium for further growth.

ELECTRICAL FUSION

In this method, which is more advantageous than the chemical fusion method, the cell membranes are manipulated through the use of an electric current. The strength of this method is that there is no possibility of toxicity to the protoplasts being fused because there are no chemicals used in this process. Besides, this method shows a considerably greater yield (about 20%) than the PEG fusion method (about 1%).

This is also a two-step process that involves first bringing the protoplasts close to each other and then disturbing the cell membranes by means of an electrical shock, which causes them to fuse together. The process of bringing the protoplasts into close physical contact is called *dielectrophoresis*. The protoplast is subjected to a low voltage oscillating sine wave current of about 1 MHz frequency. This causes the polarization of cells so that each protoplast develops a positive and negative area. When the positive and negative ends of the protoplast draw closer, we obtain the 'chain-of-pearls' appearance that is typically seen before fusion occurs. The electrical current passes along the surface of the cell membrane only and does not affect the cellular organelles. This is because the cell membrane is more conductive as compared to the cytoplasm. For successful fusion, it is important that the voltage pulse at a particular minimum threshold level is applied for a certain period. Too brief or over-extended pulses are ineffective and occasionally lethal. It is often preferred to apply multiple pulses of shorter duration as against a single long pulse.

Following protoplast fusion, culture medium is added into each well and allowed to stabilize for about an hour. The protoplasts are then subjected to centrifugation and re-suspended in the medium, followed by the usual subsequent culturing process.

13.7 SOMATIC HYBRIDIZATION

Somatic hybridization is carried out using protoplasts of two different species (inter-specific fusion) or from two diverse sources that belong to the same species. This process is carried out in four stages:

- Protoplast isolation
- Protoplast fusion
- Regeneration of plants from selected tissues
- Analysis of regenerated plants.

Somatic hybridization is an important means of generating hybrids between plants that are sexually incompatible. It can be used for the genetic modification of crops that are vegetatively propagated, species that are sterile or sub-fertile and plants which have a very long lifecycle.

Protoplast fusion leads to the generation of heterokaryons which are fusion products containing nuclei of two different genera, species or varieties. These can later turn into hybrid, totipotent cells that can give rise to plants via the process of embryogenesis or organogenesis. In the event that the two nuclear genomes are incompatible, there will be elimination of the chromosomes and in some cases, the heterokaryons so developed are unable to grow and divide further.

In some cases, there can be a recombination of mitochondrial DNA that causes the formation of fusion products with the nuclear genome of one parent in a mixed cytoplasm derived from both parents. Such fusions cause transfer of genetic elements such as chloroplasts and mitochondria that are present outside the nucleus. This leads to the transfer of the genes that are responsible for chlorophyll content, or herbicide resistance. The products of such fusion where the cytoplasm is shared are called as cytoplasmic hybrids or *cybrids*.

13.8 APPLICATIONS OF PROTOPLAST TECHNOLOGY

SEPARATION OF HYBRID CELLS

Somatic hybridization techniques permit the separation of hybrid cells developed by heterokaryotic fusion from other cells in the mixture. This technique has been used in the development of antibiotic-resistant, herbicide-resistant cell lines and cell lines with the ability to grow on specific amino acids.

This is exemplified by the somatic hybrids that have been developed from *Solanum tuberosum* which is susceptible to insects and the closely related insect-resistant wild species *Solanum chacoense*. Cell lines of *S. chacoense* contain a visible red anthocyanin but do not grow well in tissue culture and do not exhibit a regeneration of shoots. Cell lines of *S. tuberosum* cell lines do not contain anthocyanin but grow well in tissue culture, regenerating shoots readily. The cells obtained by fusing these parent cells showed an ability to grow as calli in tissue culture. Through a selection of the fast-growing calli that regenerated shoots and also contained athocyanins, it has been possible to produce a somatic hybrid variety that is insect-resistant.

GENETIC TRANSFORMATION

Genetic transformation of a single cell is possible through co-cultivation of protoplasts with *Agrobacterium tumefaciens*. This can also be achieved through the process of direct DNA transfer using polycationic chemicals, electroporation or sonication methods. In the Agrobacterium-mediated method, protoplasts are isolated and co-cultivated with *A. tumefaciens*. This is followed by an addition of antibiotics to the medium, which inhibits the bacterium's growth. Cells that undergo transformation are then grown along with the introduced gene. In cases where such Agrobacterium-mediated transformations cannot be performed, it is possible to use the direct gene transfer method that uses protoplasts to introduce beneficial genes into cereals and grasses. Through such methods, it is possible to create plants that show improved growth characteristics as well as better resistance to attack by insects and diseases.

FERTILE HYBRIDS

Protoplast fusion can be used to create fertile hybrids from sexually incompatible crosses. Such crosses that are inter-specific and inter-generic can create new plants, as shown by the example of the 'pomato' which is a cross between the tomato (*Lycopersicon esculentum*) and potato (*Solanum tuberosum*). Other reported examples include the crossing of *Datura inoxia* with *Atropa belladonna* and *Nicotiana tabacum* with *Petunia hybrida*. In these cases, however, the plants regenerated by somatic hybridization are sterile and the seeds produced are non-viable. This is evidence of the fact that protoplast fusion works best when it is restricted to plants that belong to the same genus or closely related genera.

CYBRIDS

Cybrids or cytoplasmic hybrids are cells or plants containing the nucleus of one species but cytoplasm from both the parental species. They can be formed during the course of protoplast fusion experiments due to the following reasons:

- A normal protoplast of one species fuses with an enucleate (de-activated nucleus) protoplast of the other species.
- The normal heterokaryon loses the nucleus of one of the species.
- Chromosomes of one species are slowly eliminated from the hybrid cell during mitotic division processes.

Cybrids can be produced by one of the following methods:

- Irradiation of the protoplasts belonging to one species with x-rays or γ-rays before they undergo fusion, which leads to an inactivation of their nuclei;
- Preparation of enucleate protoplasts (cytoplasts) of one species, which are then fused with normal protoplasts of another. The purpose of producing such cybrids is to combine the cytoplasmic genes of one species with the nuclear and cytoplasmic genes of another species.

This technique has been used to transfer the cytoplasmic male sterility from *Nicotiana tabacum* to *N. sylvestris* and from *Petunia hybrida* to *P. axillaris.*

13.9 TRANSGENIC PLANTS

Transgenic plants are plants that possess a gene or genes that have been transferred from a different species. Although it is possible for such DNA transfer to occur naturally, the term mainly refers to those plants that are created in vitro, using recombinant DNA methods. The purpose of such DNA transfer is to design plants that are endowed with specific characteristics that have been acquired through the artificial insertion of genes from other species and in some cases, even entirely different kingdoms.

Transgenic Bt corn, for example, which produces its own insecticide, contains a gene from a bacterium. Such plants which carry transgenes are also referred to as genetically modified or GM crops. Again, this term is used for cases where this transfer has been artificially induced, and has occurred not by the process of modification that occurs in nature over time. The natural movement of genes between species, is termed as 'horizontal' or 'lateral'gene transfer.

ADVANTAGES OF GENETICALLY ENGINEERED PLANTS

Genetically engineered plants have the following advantages:

- Longer shelf life
- Resistance to disease, herbicides, pests and non-biological stress such as drought or nitrogen starvation
- Improvement in nutritional value
- Help in the removal of pollutants from soils contaminated by organic and inorganic poisons

Creating transgenic plants

This process involves two steps.

LOCATING GENES FOR SPECIFIC TRAITS

This is presently the most difficult step where little information is available. Particular genes control factors such as yield, tolerance to stress and various other plant characteristics. Identifying the appropriate gene is important, along with an understanding of the factors that regulate that gene's expression. Moreover, it is important to know the other effects of this gene on the plant and its interaction with other genes that play an active role in the same metabolic pathway.

DESIGNING GENES FOR INSERTION

When the gene is isolated, it is cloned and subjected to several alterations prior to inserting it into plant cells. Some of these modifications are given below.

Addition of a promoter sequence that allows the gene to be correctly expressed to synthesize a protein molecule. The promoter sequence behaves as the on/off knob regulating the expression of that gene. Most promoters used until now are of the 'constitutive' type, i.e., they cause gene expression throughout the lifecycle of the plant in most tissues. The most common example of this is CaMV35S, from the cauliflower mosaic virus. Other more specific promoters show an ability to respond to changes that occur in the plant's internal or external environment. This is exemplified by the promoter from the 'cab'gene, which codes for the important chlorophyll a/b binding protein.

Modification of the cloned gene is sometimes essential to bring about better gene expression in plants. For example, the Bt gene for insect resistance shows a greater proportion of A–T nucleotide pairs compared to plants, which prefer G–C nucleotide pairs. This loophole has been bypassed through the substitution of the A–T nucleotides with G–C nucleotides in the Bt gene in a manner so as to cause minimal change in the sequence of amino acids.

Introduction of a termination sequence that signals the cellular machinery that the end of the gene sequence has been reached.

Addition of a selectable marker gene to the gene that helps with identification of plant cells or tissues that have been successful in incorporating the transgene. Selectable marker genes are chosen carefully. The commonly used genes are those that encode for certain proteins involved in antibiotic or herbicide resistance. This allows for easy identification of whether the transgene has been integrated because only such plant cells will survive when they are allowed to grow on a medium that contains the said antibiotic or herbicide. These marker genes also need to be given a promoter and termination sequence to allow their correct function.

Transforming plants

Transformation is defined as the heritable change in a cell or organism brought about by the uptake and establishment of introduced DNA. The two main methods for transforming plant cells and tissues are:

- *Gene gun method*, also known as microprojectile bombardment or biolistics, this technique has been especially useful in transforming monocot species like corn and rice.
- *Agrobacterium method*, which has been successful in dicots such as soybeans and tomatoes for many years, and is recently proving effective in monocots, too. Generally speaking, the Agrobacterium method is preferred over the gene gun, because changes are easier to monitor.
- *Viral vectors* many viruses are capable of infecting intact plant tissue, but they cannot integrate with the plant genomes. Hence, such viral vectors can be used to transfer genes and study their expression, but not for producing transgenic plants.

Agrobacterium method of plant transformation

Agrobacterium tumefaciens is a type of soil-dwelling bacteria that can infect plant cells with a piece of its own DNA, taking over the plant's cellular mechanisms and using these to proliferate. This bacterium causes crown gall disease in fruit plants.

The DNA in an *A. tumefaciens* cell is contained inside the bacterial chromosome as well as in another structure known as a Ti (tumour-inducing) plasmid. The Ti plasmid contains a stretch of DNA called T-DNA, which is the fragment responsible for the infection of plant cells. Besides, there is also a series of vir (virulence) genes which are involved in guiding the process of infection.

A. tumefaciens cannot infect intact plants, only wounded ones. A wounded plant root or stem emits some chemical signals that activate the vir genes of *A. tumefaciens*. These genes guide the further process of transferring the T-DNA contained within the Ti plasmid into the plant's chromosome. Different vir genes have different roles to play in copying the T-DNA, attaching a leader molecule, adding protective proteins all along the T-DNA strand, and opening a channel for the T-DNA to pass through the bacterial cell membrane. After the T-DNA enters the plant cell, it moves into the nucleus and gets integrated with the plant's chromosome.

When *A. tumefaciens* is to be used as a transgene vector, the tumour-inducing part of T-DNA is removed, although the T-DNA border regions and the vir genes are retained. Between the border regions, the transgene is inserted. When the T-DNA moves into the plant's nucleus, it gets incorporated into the plant's chromosomes.

Physical delivery methods or DNA-mediated gene transfer (DMGT)

The type of physical delivery method used depends on the target cell. For example,

- plasmids or DNA-loaded liposomes, or the process of electroporation is used when DNA is to be inserted into protoplasts;
- techniques such as microinjection, macroinjection or shooting with microprojectiles can be used for other explants such as organ meristems, zygotes, gametes and immature embryos.

Chemically stimulated DNA uptake by protoplasts

The most efficient way of transferring DNA into protoplasts is by using PEG. This can also help to stimulate the uptake of liposomes, and improve the efficiency of electroporation. When a 15%–25% solution of PEG is used, it leads to a precipitation of DNA, which can then be taken up by a process of endocytosis that does not cause any harm to the protoplasts. This uptake is followed by formation of the cell wall and further cell division. This method, however, shows problems in regenerating plants from the protoplasts.

Microinjection

DNA is injected into the cytoplasm or nucleus of the target cell or protoplast using glass micropipettes with 0.5–1.0 μm diameter tip. Sometimes, a specially designed micromanipulator may be used for microinjecting the DNA. This method is quite successful, but often leads to the production of chimeric plants, where only a particular part of the plant undergoes transformation. Besides, the process requires skill and is also slow and expensive.

DNA macroinjection

In this method, needles with diameters greater than the diameter of the cell are used. This method has been successful with rye, but not other cereals.

Microprojectiles (biolistics/particle gun

Heavy tungsten or gold microparticles with a diameter ranging between 1–3 μm are coated with DNA, and then accelerated to very high initial velocities in the range of 1,400 feet per second. There is a 'bullet' to carry these microprojectiles and push them into living plant cells. This bullet is required to help the microparticles penetrate the cell walls of intact tissue.

The process uses an explosive charge (cordite explosion) or shock waves to accelerate the microprojectiles. It has been successful in transfer of soybean, tobacco, maize, rice and wheat. This is one of the most advantageous methods because multiple hits occur simultaneously, increasing the probability of successful transfer. Since intact cells of all types, size and shape can be used, none of the difficulties seen with protoplasts are present.

Electroporation

This method depends on the use of short electrical impulses of high field strength to make the protoplast more permeable to DNA transfer. However, it suffers from drawbacks similar to the methods that use protoplasts.

Selection and regeneration

After the process of gene insertion, plant tissues are transferred into a selective medium prepared with an antibiotic or herbicide. As a result, only those plants which succeed in expressing the selectable marker gene will survive. The fact that they survive is proof that they have incorporated the transgene.

Through tissue culture, plantlets are generated and allowed to grow into whole plants. After these plants produce seeds, further generations of plants that develop from these modified parent plants are evaluated for expression of the trait.

Plant breeding and testing

Before transgenic plants can be produced on a large scale, there has to be extensive evaluation to study the effect of the new gene on other properties of the plant as well as on the ecosystem. Such transgenic plants are monitored throughout their lifecycle to study the activity of the newly introduced gene and its manner of transmission to the next generation. The growth of the plant, the yield of crop or fruit and the quality of the produce is evaluated constantly until there is sufficient evidence to justify its breeding on a larger scale. However, such plants are not bred in isolation, but by crossing them with improved existing crop varieties. This is significant as no genetic transfer can transform all the qualities of a plant to the desired levels. Hence, repeated crossing with good varieties is imperative to imbue the plant with all the desirable properties. After crossing with improved varieties, the new variety is also crossed several times with the improved parent plant, and this process is called *backcrossing*. This is done to ensure that the maximum amount of the improved parent's genome is recovered to coexist with the newly introduced transgene. After this backcrossing is completed, multi-location evaluation trials are performed over several years by breeding the plants in greenhouses as well as the field to study the transgene's effects on the environment.

Objections to transgenic plants

Various doubts have been raised regarding the safety of transgenic or genetically modified plants. A few of these are discussed here.

Effect on human health
The fact that antibiotic resistance markers are used during the development of transgenic crops implies that the new variety contains the DNA that codes for resistance to these antibiotics. This has raised fears that transgenic foods can induce antibiotic resistance. However, there has not yet been any report of incidents of antibiotic resistance arising from the DNA in transgenic crops.

Effect on nutritional quality
Considering that many genetically engineered foods claim to have higher nutritional quality than conventional foods, it is important that thorough research be conducted to prove this. Most existing evidence suggests that genetically modified foods have nutritional levels that are similar to those in natural foods.

Effect on the environment
One of the major concerns with transgenic plants is that they contain a gene for herbicide resistance which can pass on to weeds growing nearby through natural hybridization processes. Such an event can lead to weeds developing resistance to commonly used herbicides, and prove dangerous in the long run.

13.10 IMMOBILIZATION OF PLANT CELLS

Immobilization is defined as the imprisonment of biocatalyst or cells in a distinct phase that allows exchange with, but is separated from a bulk phase, in which the substrates, effector or inhibitor are dispersed and monitored.

It is the newest culture technology for plant cells in which cells are encouraged to grow together in a multi-cellular, partially organized condition. When such cells are allowed to remain static, it leads to the development of physical and chemical gradients which mimic the natural environment of plants.

Immobilization has the following advantages:

- Immobilization facilitates the use of continuous flow processes.
- Plant cells can be reused.
- Cell content that is induced by immobilization can help in the production of important secondary metabolites.
- Immobilization prevents the harmful effects of shear forces on the delicate plant cells.

Why plant cell immobilization?

Studies carried out on cell differentiation processes show that there is a definite relationship between the morphological organization of cells and the level of cytodifferentiation, which in turn influences the rate of growth of cultures. Culture growth rate plays a major role in the synthesis and accumulation of secondary metabolites. A few examples are shown below.

- Cell cultures of many solanaceous species show a higher accumulation of alkaloid within partially organized cells as compared with cells that grow rapidly and are more loosely associated.
- Aggregation has been found to play a role in the regulation of anthocyanin synthesis in carrot culture.
- In *Populus alba*, it has been shown that aggregated culture cells produce glycosylating salicylic acid with greater efficiency than cells which are freely suspended in the medium.

Another factor to consider is that primary and secondary pathways are always in competition. So, under conditions that are conducive for rapid growth and division, there will be greater production of primary metabolites like proteins. However, when conditions cause slowing down of growth, then the same precursor will produce secondary metabolites such as phenolics or alkaloids. This is the reason why it is believed that immobilized cells, where growth is slower, are better suited for the production of secondary metabolites.

Methods of immobilization

Gel entrapment

It is the most common method used. Calcium alginate is the gel used. A mixture of sodium alginate and the cell is extruded drop-wise into a $CaCl_2$ solution, leading to immediate hardening of the cells into beads. Alginate is the preferred gel because of its mildness and easy handling. Moreover, it can have beneficial effects on the production of secondary metabolites. For example, a three-fold increase has been observed in the production of ajmalicine by immobilizing *Catharanthus roseus* cells in calcium alginate and a 250% increase of shikonin production is shown by immobilizing *Lithospermum erythrorhizon* cells in calcium alginate.

BIOFILM

Gels are used as a support in the formation of biofilm. For example, *Catharanthus roseus* cells are grown on the surface of calcium alginate beads present within the interspatial volume of a packed column. The cells showed some growth and there was an increase in the alkaloid content of the medium.

ADSORPTION

Plant cells are immobilized by adsorption to various support materials such as fibre glass, polystyrene, sulphonated polystyrene and fluorinated ether. Factors that play an important role include the surface tension of the cells, the surface and the culture liquid. Culture age is important to obtain good adsorption. It has been found that adsorption is best when cells have reached the age of 8–14 days, probably because there is a greater secretion of polysaccharides by the cells at this time.

FOAM IMMOBILIZATION

This method uses polyurethane foam, and is a very simple immobilization method because the cells migrate into the foam without any force. Hence, there is no requirement for high temperature or ionic strength, which can influence the viability of the cells. The foam can be used in various forms—as cubes, attached to stainless steel wire or wound sheets or tubes. One of the disadvantages of this method is that it usually takes about 10–15 days for all the cells to be immobilized in the foam. It has also been observed that the effects of the immobilization in polyurethane foam are not uniform for all cell cultures.

The equipment used are described below.

Flat-bed bioreactors

It is the simplest system in which cells are loaded on a substratum of polypropylene fabric held in a glass vessel. Liquid nutrient medium that is supplied from a reservoir set above the culture vessel constantly drips on the fabric and moves across by capillary action to feed the cells. Liquid medium is removed from the vessel by using a peristaltic pump and returned to the reservoir. The rate of supply of medium in the culture vessel is controlled by the rate at which it is pumped back into the reservoir. This technique provides cell to cell contact and sequential chemical treatments on the stationary culture.

Column reactors

It is a modification of the flatbed bioreactor in vertical mode. It has the advantage that it provides better control over the supply of nutrients, saves space and caters to the need of scaling up to an industrial scale. Here, the culture vessel is a vertical glass column through which the nutrient medium is circulated before being pumped back into the reservoir. The column is supported with the inert matrix along the length to prevent settling of the cells at the bottom of the column.

Applications of immobilization techniques

- It enables large-scale production of secondary metabolites.
- It increases the shelf life for long-term storage or transport of cells and protoplasts.
- It is valuable in studying the biochemical response of plant cells to infection.
- It is helpful in the developmental studies of cells, protoplasts and cell metabolism.

SUMMARY

- Protoplasts (plant cells without cell wall) are isolated and purified and then used for preparing genetically modified organisms.
- Transgenic plants are those plants with a gene transferred from another species to impart specific desirable characteristics. Many methods can be used for the formation of transgenic plants such as DNA mediated gene transfer and viral vectors.
- The common distrust of transgenic plants arises due to the dangers of antibiotic resistance, damage to the environment and gene flow from crop to weed.
- Plant cells can be immobilized by adsorbing them on some solid surface or entrapment within a medium and such immobilized enzymes have many advantages, especially in the production of secondary metabolites.

Exercises

Long answers

1. What are the different techniques of protoplast fusion?
2. What are transgenic plants? Explain the process with an example.

Short answers

3. Explain gene transfer using viral vectors.
4. What are the limitations of transgenic plants?
5. Explain immobilization of plant cells.
6. Explain the role of *Agrobacterum tumefaciens* in transgenic plant production.

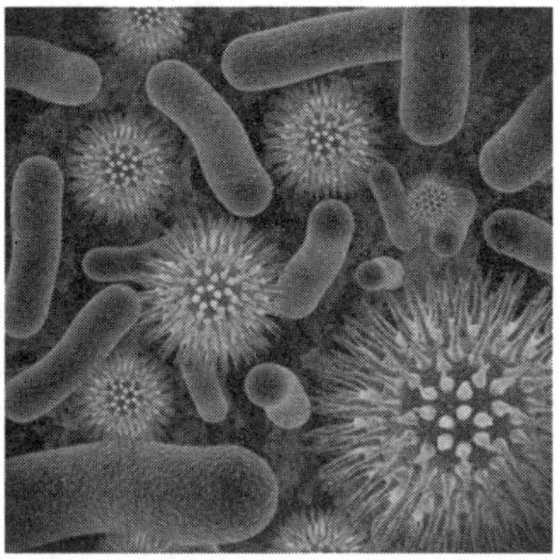

14

Enzyme Biotechnology

In This Chapter, You Will Learn

- The steps involved in the extraction of enzymes from their source
- The techniques for purification of isolated enzymes
- The techniques, advantages and disadvantages of immobilization of enzymes
- The applications of immobilized enzymes

Enzymes are colloidal, proteinaceous compounds that can be extracted from living tissues, and purified for further use. A purified enzyme can be used to catalyze a specific biochemical reaction outside the cells. Enzymes can also be altered for a variety of purposes, using techniques such as enzyme modelling and gene manipulation. In the pharmaceutical industry, enzyme engineering is rapidly growing to be an innovative method for developing new biotechnology-based products. Enzymatic reactions have a distinct advantage over chemical reactions because they occur under milder conditions, are faster, and highly specific.

14.1 ISOLATION OF ENZYMES

All enzymes possess well-defined physicochemical organization; this ordering is highly sensitive to changes in external conditions. The smallest of changes in the chemical composition can significantly alter enzyme activity, and may even lead to total inactivation. Therefore, during the process of isolation, purification and processing of enzymes, great care is required. All these procedures have to be performed under controlled conditions of pH, ionic strength and temperature. The extraction and purification processes for enzymes are similar to those used for proteins, with the only difference being the need to assay the enzyme at every step of the process to confirm the retention of activity. There are four main steps through which enzyme processing is done:

- Extraction
- Preparation
- Purification
- Final processing of the enzyme

Extraction of enzymes

An extraction medium such as a buffer is mixed with the fresh tissue that contains the enzyme, and the tissue is crushed into a paste by using a mortar-pestle, homogenizer, sonicator or blender. Controlled temperature conditions are required to carry out this operation because enzymes get inactivated at higher temperatures. Generally, a temperature range of 0–4°C is used.

Both the molarity as well as pH of the extraction medium should be adjusted to achieve maximum solubility and activity of the enzyme. Most extraction media incorporate EDTA as one of the ingredients to remove heavy metals which may lead to an inhibition of enzyme activity. Besides, EDTA also facilitates the release of enzymes from within cells by causing disruption of the cell membrane and membranes of cell organelles. Often, detergents are used for solubilizing membranes; Triton-X is a typical example.

Thiols such as mercaptoethanol are added to the extraction medium. These compounds serve to maintain the sulphydryl bond of the enzymes which may be broken during extraction. After completion of the extraction process, the extract is filtered to remove cell debris and fibres that often appear in the final extraction product.

Preparation of crude enzymes

Centrifugation

The filtered enzyme extract is subjected to centrifugation to remove any remaining cell debris, cell organelles and other molecular aggregates. Besides assisting in purification of the enzymes, this step also helps in characterizing them. Enzymes move through the extract solution at a particular rate and occupy a specific position within the centrifuge tube, depending on their mass and shape.

Precipitation

Enzymes carry an ionic charge and hence, can be precipitated through the use of certain neutralizing chemicals that also carry charge. When enzyme charge is broken, it leads to an aggregation of the enzyme molecules, causing them to sediment at the bottom of the container as a precipitate. The use of an acid, base or any other compound can lead to a precipitation of the enzyme, provided the pH reaches the isoelectric pH of the enzyme. The *isoelectric pH* is that pH at which the enzyme carries an equal number of positive and negative charges and is least soluble. However, the use of acids and bases can cause inactivation of enzymes and hence, this method is not generally used.

The process of 'salting out' using compounds such as ammonium sulphate is an alternative to precipitation using acids and bases. These salts bring about a change in solvent structure, which in turn leads to a corresponding change in the protein conformation. Moreover, when the salt competes with the proteins for the limited number of solvent molecules available, it causes precipitation because the salt has a greater affinity for solvent as compared to the protein. Ammonium sulphate, although highly effective, is not much used today because of its corrosive nature and the fact that it releases toxic ammonia at higher temperatures.

Certain organic solvents such as acetone, methanol and ethanol which are miscible with water, can also be used for precipitating enzymes from solution. These solvents act to reduce the solubility of the proteins, causing their precipitation. They have to be cooled to a temperature of 4–6°C before use. Precipitation is then carried out at 0°C since precipitation at room temperature causes denaturation of enzymes. Care should be taken to avoid high local concentrations of the solvents. An effective way of doing this is to add the solvents slowly and in drops, to avoid high local concentration.

Non-ionic polymers such as polyethylene glycol (PEG), alginates, pectates, carboxy methyl cellulose (CMC), polyacrylic and polymeta-acrylic acids, which are water soluble are also used to purify enzymes.

Purification of enzymes

Any one of the following three methods can be used for purification: (i) dialysis, (ii) chromatography or (iii) electrophoresis.

Dialysis

This technique helps in the removal of small molecules from the enzyme. The enzyme precipitate is mixed with the same buffer solution that was used for its extraction. This solution is kept inside a dialysis bag that is generally constructed of cellophane and securely sealed. This bag is suspended in a vessel containing either distilled water or a buffer of known molarity and ionic composition. Occasionally, some other salts or chemicals may also be added to this liquid to prevent inactivation of the enzyme. This solution needs to be replenished with fresh solution at regular intervals during the course of the dialysis.

CHROMATOGRAPHY

This is the most common method used in the purification of enzymes. Four techniques of chromatography can be adopted including gel filtration, adsorption, ion exchange and affinity.

Gel filtration chromatography

In gel filtration chromatography, enzyme molecules are segregated based on their molecular size. Hence, it is also known as *molecular exclusion* or *molecular sieve chromatography*.

The basic arrangement for gel filtration chromatography is similar to that for adsorption chromatography. A column of glass or steel is packed with a gel—generally, Sephadex gel—that is composed of a cross-linked dextran obtained from a variety of bacteria. Various grades of Sephadex such as G-10, G-30, G-50, G-100, G-150, and G-200 are available, which differ in their pore size. When the enzyme solution is poured on top of the column, the various components move down the column and are segregated on the basis of their molecular sizes. Larger molecules are eluted first from the column, with the elution volume being logarithmically proportional to the molecular size.

Adsorption chromatography

In this method, the enzyme solution is allowed to flow through a column containing some inert material packed within a glass or steel tube. The column packing is generally made up of fine particles of adsorbents such as silica, charcoal, alumina, calcium phosphate, and hydroxyapatite among others. As the solution elutes, it is collected in small fractions. The content of each fraction is estimated by measuring the absorption at 280 nm using a UV spectrophotometer. This technique is commonly used in the separation of enzymes such as basic and acidic RNase, acidic DNase, phosphodiesterase or phosphomonoesterase.

Ion exchange chromatography

Ion exchange resins have high capacities and are therefore very useful in the purification and concentration of proteins. When the pH of the solution is varied, it changes the net charge on the enzymes, and this causes an alteration in the strength of their adsorption to the resin. Thus, an enzyme which is initially tightly held on the exchange resin can be separated by changing the pH or ionic strength or both.

Affinity chromatography

This method depends on the use of an insoluble ligand of the enzyme such as a substrate, an inhibitor, or a cofactor. There are particular forces of attraction due to which sorption occurs. The use of such sorbents allows better and more selective isolation of pure enzymes from various sources.

Electrophoresis

This method of separation depends on the movement of particles suspended in a liquid under the influence of a uniform electric field. Since enzymes bear a specific charge, they can be separated from other components of the extract through the use of this technique.

Final processing of enzymes

After purification, the enzyme extract is concentrated and subjected to sterilization by filtration in order to remove the microbial contamination that may be present. The enzyme is then freeze dried in the presence of other additives such as dextrans or sugar substrates.

14.2 IMMOBILIZATION OF ENZYMES

Immobilized enzymes are enzymes that are anchored to an inert material in order to modify their stability and other properties. Immobilization is especially important in industrial applications of enzymes. Industrial use of enzymes is expensive because of various shortcomings. When an enzyme catalyzed reaction reaches its end point, there is a need to separate the unchanged enzyme from the final product mixture. Separation, purification and recovery of intact enzymes are often time consuming and expensive processes. Immobilizing the enzymes allows faster and better recovery, thus reducing overall costs.

Definition
Immobilization is defined as the arrest of a biocatalyst or cells in a distinct phase that allows exchange with, but is separated from a bulk phase, in which the substrates, effector or inhibitor are dispersed and monitored.

Methods of immobilization

Whatever may be the method used for immobilizing enzymes, great care is required to ensure that sufficiently mild conditions are used to prevent denaturation of the enzyme. This is critical because denaturation due to heat or pH changes can lead to a loss of the tertiary and quaternary level structures of the enzyme that are essential for enzyme action.

Broadly, two types of methods are used:

- On-surface immobilization
- Within-surface immobilization

On-surface immobilization

Three main types of techniques are used—covalent coupling, adsorption and complexation or chelation.

Covalent coupling

An enzyme can bind covalently with inert support materials by any of the following two mechanisms:

- Through reactive grooves which are present on the side chains of lysine, asparagine, tyrosine, aspartic acid, histidine, cysteine, serine, glutamic acid and other amino acids
- At the terminal amino or carboxyl groups present on the enzyme molecule.

For effective coupling between the inert support and the enzyme, the former is activated by treating it with certain activators. However, caution is required during this step because there is a possibility of the active sites of the enzyme getting coupled with the support material, leading to a loss of the enzyme's activity.

Adsorption

In this method, enzymes are attached to the inert support material through adsorption. The inert support may be either charged or neutral. This is one of the simplest and most economical methods of immobilizing enzymes. This process involves allowing the enzyme and polymer support to interact in a tank reactor with constant stirring. Alternatively, it is possible to allow the enzyme to percolate through a packed bed of the support material within a tube or column.

- Physical adsorption involves hydrophobic interactions between enzyme and support material. However, the bonding is not very reliable since minor variations in pH and ionic strength of the solution in which it is immersed may cause the enzyme to leak from the support.
- Chemical adsorption involves the formation of ionic, hydrogen, covalent or hydrophobic bonds, or a combination of all of them. However, ionic bonds have disadvantages that are similar to those of physical adsorption.

The best polymer adsorbent is one that leads to strong bond formation, with minimal chances of inactivation. Alumina, calcium phosphate, Amberlite, CMC, Bentonite and Sephadex are a few examples of adsorbent materials that can be used. Some enzymes and their support materials are listed in Table 14.1.

Complexation or *chelation*

It can be done by two mechanisms. One is the formation of chloroaqua complexes of titanium in HCl solution. The other involves the formation of hydrous transition metal oxide complexes. Metals such as cobalt, manganese, zinc, copper, tin and chromium are commonly used in this process. The process of complexation is advantageous because it does not require any chemical derivatization nor activation of the support material.

Table 14.1 Common support materials used for adsorption

Enzyme	Support material
Covalent coupling	
Aminoglycosidase	DEAE cellulose
Cellulose pectinase	Polyurethane
Glucose isomerase	Polyurethane
Glucose oxidase	Porous glass
Adsorption	
Catalase/invertase	Calcium phosphate
α-Amylase	Calcium phosphate
Glucose oxidase	Cellophane

WITHIN-SURFACE IMMOBILIZATION

This is a process in which the enzyme is trapped or encapsulated within a matrix consisting of a polymer with a high degree of cross-linking or within microcapsules or distributed in a distinct non-aqueous phase. The lack of points of attachment of enzyme to matrix ensures that there is no chance of a stearic blockage as is commonly observed in covalent bonding.

Entrapment

A gel or polymer may be used for entrapment in the following ways.

IN SITU POLYMERIZATION AS HYDROGEL This is the most preferred method since such gels form highly stable complexes with the enzyme. Since they are easily wetted, they provide better access of substrates to the enzyme.

In this process, the enzyme is dispersed or dissolved in an aqueous buffer that contains acrylamide with bisacrylate compounds serving as the cross-linking agent. The concentration of acrylamide plays a crucial role in determining the gel strength. Besides acrylamide, other monomers can also be used to form gels. These include bi-functional acrylates like PEG –dimethacrylate and hydroxyl ethyl methacrylate (HEMA).

POLYCONDENSATION REACTION Enzymes can be immobilized by entrapping them at the points of cross-linkage between polymers during their condensation. This is exemplified by the use of bis-isocynates with polyalcohols or polyamines. The product formed consists of urethanes where the enzyme is held by cross-linking with bi-functional glutaraldehyde.

GELATIN GELS Gelatin is a highly hydrophilic protein with strong swelling power, making it a good candidate for gel formation. A 10% w/v gelatin aqueous solution is kept at a temperature of around 30–40°C. A 20% w/v formaldehyde solution or a 50% v/v alcohol solution is added to allow it to harden. Enzymes are dispersed in de-mineralized water and added slowly into this viscous liquid. This is immediately transferred into a cylindrical mould, and allowed to set into a gel by maintaining at 25°C for four hours. The temperature is then allowed to increase gradually to room temperature, and the gel is cut into thin discs with a thickness of 0.2–0.4 cm.

Encapsulation

Emulsions, microcapsules, dehydrated, rehydrated vesicles (DRVs) and Reverse phase evaporation methods are commonly used for encapsulation.

EMULSIONS A multiple emulsion system of the w/o/w type is stabilized by detergents. This emulsion system can be used to immobilize the enzymes, and keep them separate from the bulk fluids.

MICROCAPSULES Micron-sized spherical particles are formed, in which a liquid or suspension is entrapped in a semi-permeable membrane. This method is used for the immobilization of biocatalysts or gels. The microcapsules can be formed either by using membrane reactors or membrane hardening agents. The membrane reactor method uses compounds such as cellulose acetates, polyamides and polysulphones. Hardening agents used include ethyl cellulose, polyesters, cellulose acetates, cellulose diacetate and eudragits.

DEHYDRATED REHYDRATED VESICLES (DRVS) To prepare the DRVs, a hydrated fluid of enzymes is made and frozen. This is followed by rehydration using plain phosphate saline buffer. The higher the concentration of NaCl or KCl, the greater the rate of entrapment. However, an increase in sugar concentration leads to decrease in entrapment.

REVERSE PHASE EVAPORATION METHOD In this method, a water-in-oil emulsion is prepared first and this is subjected to phase reversal by the solvent evaporation method. The emulsion is then sonicated and dried using a rotary evaporator under vacuum.

REVERSE MICELLES They are the association colloids of surfactants in organic solvents. Enzymes can be subjected to entrapment within such micelles in which the polar ends of the surfactants get oriented towards the aqueous enzymatic phase. This is the method of choice in conditions where the enzyme could be denatured due to reaction with organic solvents. In fact, this method has been successfully used with enzymes such as α-amylase, invertase and arginase.

Advantages of immobilization

1. Immobilized enzymes show greater stability because they are bound to a matrix, rendering them more resistant to variations in reaction conditions such as pH or temperature.
2. It allows the localization of enzymes to a particular area. This increases the efficiency of their action and also makes for easier separation and recovery of the enzyme.

3. Immobilized enzymes can be packed within columns, allowing their use over prolonged periods.
4. There is less loss of enzyme during the process of recovery and hence, the same batch of enzyme can be used repeatedly over multiple reactions.
5. The ease of recovery and ability to reuse the enzymes makes the process an economical one.
6. Certain manipulations that are impossible with free enzymes can be easily achieved with immobilized ones. For example, a reaction can be stopped within minutes by simply removing the enzyme from the reaction mixture.
7. Thermal stability of immobilized enzymes is greater and hence, it is possible to use higher temperatures to further increase the rate of reaction.

Disadvantages of immobilization

1. It is an expensive process.
2. If the active sites of the enzymes are bound in the matrix or get occluded during the process of adsorption, the enzyme activity is reduced or inactivated completely.
3. Immobilization is not possible in those reactions where the substrate is insoluble in water.

Applications of enzyme immobilization

Immobilized enzymes were first used for industrial purposes in the resolution of racemic mixtures of amino acids that were synthesized in the laboratory. The Tanabe Seiyaku Company of Japan used the enzyme amino acid acylase in immobilized form by binding it through ionic interaction with Sephadex. Now, immobilized enzymes are used in a variety of industrial applications as discussed below.

INDUSTRIAL APPLICATIONS

The main industrial applications are:

1. Glucose syrup is converted to high fructose syrup through the use of glucose isomerase enzyme. This is predominantly seen in non-tropical countries with vast reserves of starch material. In tropical countries, immobilized invertase enzyme is used to hydrolyze sucrose obtained from sugarcane to form high fructose syrup.
2. Fumaric acid is converted to L-aspartic acid by the action of aspartase enzyme using immobilized whole cells of *E. coli*.
3. Immobilized enzymes are widely used in the dairy industry to convert milk into a lactose-hydrolyzed form for use by lactose-intolerant individuals. This process is achieved through the use of immobilized β-galactosidase enzyme.

4. In the pharmaceutical industry, immobilized enzymes are used in the synthesis of 6-aminopenicillanic acid (6-APA) through deacylation of the side chain of Penicillin G or V, by the action of penicillin acylase enzyme.
5. Immobilized oxidoreductases are used widely in synthetic transformations such as those involved in the asymmetric synthesis of amino acids, steroids and other pharmaceutical compounds.
6. Catalase in immobilized form is used to destroy hydrogen peroxide which is the chemical used in the cold sterilization of milk.
7. Production of acids has shown greater yield when immobilized enzyme is used. A good example is the formation of acetic acid using immobilized *Acetobacter aceti*.

Analytical Applications

1. Immobilized enzymes are useful in analytical biochemistry as biosensors. These are constructed as enzyme electrodes to allow the continuous monitoring of small concentrations of particular biochemical entities. The use of a urea electrode is an example.
2. In clinical chemistry analyses, immobilized enzymes are used in thermistors to measure the amount of heat generated during an enzymatic reaction.

SUMMARY

- Purified enzymes can be used in specific biochemical reactions outside the cells.
- The preparation of enzymes includes processes of precipitation, centrifugation and purification.
- Purification of enzymes can be done by dialysis, chromatography and electrophoresis methods.
- Enzymes used industrially have a few drawbacks such as instability, high costs of isolation, high costs of purification and recovery. To overcome these problems, enzymes are immobilized.
- Immobilization refers to the arrest of biocatalyst or cells in a distinct phase that allows exchange with, but is separated from a bulk phase, in which the substrates, effector or inhibitor are dispersed and monitored.
- Entrapment and encapsulation methods are used for immobilizing enzymes.
- Immobilized enzymes are used for various applications like preparation of lactose-hydrolysed milk, resolution of racemic mixtures, synthetic biotransformations, cold sterilization of milk, and as biosensors.

Exercises

Long answers

1. Define the term 'enzyme' and list the important properties of enzymes.
2. Describe in detail the techniques of isolation and purification of enzymes.

Short answers

3. What are the advantages and disadvantages of immobilized enzymes?
4. What are the different methods of immobilizing enzymes?
5. What are the main applications of immobilized enzymes?

Bibliography

General

Agrawal SS and Paridhavi M, *Herbal Drug Technology*, Universities Press, Hyderabad, 2007.

Agrawal SS, Tamrakar BP, Paridhavi M, *Clinically Useful Herbal Drugs*, Ahuja Publishing House, 2005.

Chaudhri RD, *Herbal Drugs Industry*, Eastern Publishers, 2006.

Divakar CM, *Plant Drug Evaluation*, M/s CD Remedies, Kerala, 2002.

Gupta PK, *Elements of Biotechnology*, Rastogi Publications, 1997.

Herbal Pharmacopoeia of India, Government of India, Ministry of Health, Revised edition, 2002.

Kalia AN, *Textbook of Industrial Pharmacognosy*, CBS Publishers, Delhi, 2007.

Kokate CK, Purohit AP and Gokhale SB. *Pharmacognosy*, Nirali Prakashan, Pune, 2008.

Prajapati ND, Purohit SS, Sharma K Arun, Tarun Kumar, *A Handbook of Medicinal Plants—A Complete Source Book*, Agrobios (India), 2003.

Rangari Vinod D, Pharmacognosy and Phytochemistry, Part 2, Career Publications, Nashik, 2003.

Wikipedia, Ayurveda; available at en.wikipedia.org/wiki/Ayurveda

Chapter 1 Herbal Drug Industry

Anon P, 1988, Pharmaceutical and cosmetic compositions containing tomato plant extracts for the treatment of skin diseases, Patent-Israel, 78 (820),15.

Business Maps of India, Pharmaceutical Companies in India, 25 October 2010; available at *http://business.mapsofindia.com/india-company/pharmaceutical.html,* *http://www.pharmabiz.com/article/detnews.asp?articleid=25018 Exsectionid=50*

Joshi K, Indian Herbal Sector, *India Science and Technology*, 2008; available at SSRN: http://ssrn.com/abstract=1474143

Kobayashi S, Effects of harvesting impacts and rehabilitation of tropical rain forest, *Journal of Plant Research*, 99–106, 1994.

Mehtaa VA, *Indian Herbal Drug Industry—Future Prospects*, 2004,

National Medicinal Plants Board, Government of India, *http://nmpb.nic.in/index.php*

Polshettiwar SA, Ayurveda emphasis relationship between man and plants throughout the development of human culture; available at *http://www.pharmainfo.net/reviews/indian-herbal-drug-industry-future-prospects-review*

Robbers JE and Tyler VE, *Tyler's Herbs of Choice*, CBS Publishers, Delhi, 2002.

Chapter 2 Patents

Bellis M, Plant Patents: What is a plant patent? What does it mean to invent a plant? available at *http://inventors.about.com/cs/biopatents/a/aa_plant_patent.htm*

Can IP rights protect plants? available at *http://www.patentlens.net/daisy/bios/1234.html*

European Federation of Biotechnology: Task Group on Public Perceptions of Biotechnology, Patenting in Biotechnology; available at *http://www.efb-central.org/images/uploads/Patenting_in_Biotechnology_English.pdf*

Good News India, Abduction of Turmeric provokes India's wrath: The war to rescue neem, turmeric and other goddesses of India's bio-diversity from knowledge pirates, 15 September 2002; available at *http://www.goodnewsindia.com/Pages/content/traditions/turmeric.html*

Intellectual Property Office: Types of IP; available at *http://ns3.patent.gov.uk/types.htm*

Ramesh Randeep, India moves to protect traditional medicines from foreign patents: India fights to protect ancient treatments from western pharmaceutical companies, 22 February 2009; available at *http://www.guardian.co.uk/world/2009/feb/22/india-protect-traditional-medicines*

Traditional Knowledge Digital Library; available at *http://www.tkdl.res.in/tkdl/langdefault/common/Home.asp?GL=Eng*

United States Patent and Trademark Office, Patents; available at *http://www.uspto.gov/inventors/patents.jsp*

Vasudeva PK, Patenting Biotech Products: Complex Issues; available at *http://www.jstor.org/pss/4409857* Wikipedia, Plant breeders' rights; available at *http://en.wikipedia.org/wiki/Plant_breeders'_rights*

World Intellectual Property Organization, Using Traditional Knowledge to Revive the Body and a Community; available at *http://www.wipo.int/ipadvantage/en/details.jsp?id=2599*

World Intellectual Property Organization, What is Intellectual Property Right? Available at *http://www.wipo.int/about-ip/en*

www.worldbank.org/afr/.../Benefit_Sharing-Kani_Tribe_Model.ppt

Chapter 3 Standardization of Herbal Drugs

Bandaranayake WM., Quality Control, Screening, Toxicity, and Regulation of Herbal Drugs; available at *http://faculty.ksu.edu.sa/23494/Documents/Quality%20Control%20of%20Herbal%20Drugs.pdf*

Eric Brand, Are You Using the Correct Fang Ji?; available at http://www.bluepoppy.com/blog/blogs/blog1.php/2010/01/08/mixed-fangji-jpg

Inamdar N, Edalat S, Kotwal VB and Pawar S, Herbal drugs in milieu of modern drugs. *Int J Green Pharm* (online serial), 2:2-8, 2008. Available from: *http://www.greenpharmacy.info/text.asp?2008/2/1/2/39154*

Sapna Shrikumar, Uma Maheswari M, Suganthi A and Ravi TK, WHO guidelines for herbal drug standardization, *Pharma Info*; available at *http://www.pharmainfo.net/reviews/who-guidelines-herbal-drug-standardization*

Chapter 4 Traditional Systems of Medicine

Acupuncture: The Conceptual Basis of Traditional Chinese Medicine; available at *http://www.healthy.net/scr/article.aspx?Id=1278*

Aromaweb: Aromatherapy and Essential Oils; available at *http://www.aromaweb.com/*

Choudhary Ranjit Roy and Uton Muchtar Rafei, (Eds), *Traditional Medicine in Asia, WHO, 2002.*

Holistic Online: Ayurveda; available at *http://www.holisticonline.com/ayurveda/ayv_home.html*

Holistic Online: Homeopathy; available at *http://www.holistic-online.com/homeopathy/homeo_principles.html*

Siddha System of Medicine: About Siddha Systems of Medicine; available at *http://www.sysindia.com/medical/aboutsiddha.html*

Understanding Chinese Medicine: What is it?; available at *http://www.docmisha.com/understanding/what.htm*

University of Maryland Medical Center: Ayurveda; available at *http://www.umm.edu/altmed/articles/ayurveda-000348.html*

Chapter 5 Ayurvedic Formulations

Nadkarni AK, *Indian Materia Medica*, Vols 1 and 2, Popular Prakashan Pvt. Ltd, Mumbai.

Chapter 6 Traditional Drugs

ICS Unido, Asparagus racemosus Willd; available at http://portal.ics.trieste.it/MAPs/MedicinalPlants_Plant.aspx?id=581

Chapter 7 Isolation of Compounds from Natural Sources

Peach K and Tracey MV, *Modern Methods of Plant Analysis*, Vols 1–7, Springer and Verlag, Berlin, 1955.

Chapter 9 Enzymes

Description of some enzymes used in therapy; available at http://www.enzymetherapy.at/cms/?page_id=8

Papain production, Practical Action; available at http://practicalaction.org/docs/technical_information_service/papain.pdf

Chapter 10 Nutraceuticals

Kalra EK, Nutraceutical—Definition and Introduction, *AAPS PharmSci.*, 5 (2), article 25, 2003; available at http://www.aapsj.org/view.asp?art=ps050325

Nutraceuticals, North Carolina Association for Biomedical Research; available at http://www.aboutbioscience.org/pdfs/Nutraceuticals.pdf

Omega-3 fatty acids, fish oil, alpha-linolenic acid, Mayo Clinic; available at http://www.mayoclinic.com/health/fish-oil/NS_patient-fishoil

Spirulina, University of Maryland Medical Center; available at http://www.umm.edu/altmed/articles/spirulina-000327.htm

What are Functional Foods and Nutraceuticals? Agriculture and Agri-Food Canada; available at http://www4.agr.gc.ca/AAFC-AAC/display-afficher.do?id=1171305207040&lang=eng

Chapter 11 Polyploidy

Adams KL and Wendel JF, Polyploidy and genome evolution in plants, *Science Direct*; available at http://www.eeob.iastate.edu/faculty/WendelJ/pdfs/Adams_and_Wende_COPB_2005.pdf

John K, *Polyploidy in plants*, West Virginia University, Eberly College of Arts and Sciences; available at http://www.as.wvu.edu/~kgarbutt/QuantGen/Gen535_2_2004/Polyploidy.html

Polyploidy, Kimball's Biology Pages; available at http://users.rcn.com/jkimball.ma.ultranet/BiologyPages/P/Polyploidy.html

Woodhouse M, Burkart-Waco D and Comai L, Polyploidy, *Nature Education*, 2(1), 2009; available at http://www.nature.com/scitable/topicpage/polyploidy-1552814

Chapter 12 Plant Biotechnology

Gupta PK, *Elements of Biotechnology*, Rastogi Publications, 1997.

http://nsdl.niscair.res.in/bitstream/123456789/668/1/revised+introduction+to+plant+biotechnology.pdf

Pighin J, Your guide to plant cell culture, *The Science Creative Quarterly*; available at http://www.scq.ubc.ca/your-guide-to-plant-cell-culture/

Rhitu Rai, *Genetics and Plant Breeding: Introduction to Plant Biotechnology*, National Research Centre on Plant Biotechnology; available at

Trigiano RN and Gray DJ, *Plant Tissue Concepts and Laboratory Exercises*, (Eds), CRC Press; available at http://pages.towson.edu/jsaunder/Saunders%20Publications/60.Use%20of%20protoplasts%20for%20plant%20improvement.pdf

Types of culture, Biotechnology 4 U; available at http://www.biotechnology4u.com/plant_biotechnology_types_culture.html

Chapter 13 Protoplast Technology

Gupta PK, Elements of Biotechnology, Rastogi Publications, 1997.

Immobilization of enzymes or whole cells; available at http://www.molecular-plant-biotechnology.info/enzyme-biotechnology/immobilization-of-enzymes-OR-whole-cells.htm

Pighin J, Your guide to plant cell culture, *The Science Creative Quarterly*; available at http://www.scq.ubc.ca/your-guide-to-plant-cell-culture

Ritu Rai, *Genetics and plant breeding: Introduction to plant biotechnology*, National Research Centre on Plant Biotechnology; available at http://nsdl.niscair.res.in/bitstream/123456789/668/1/revised+introduction+to+plant+biotechnology.pdf

Transformation systems, Plants in action, Edition 1; available at http://plantsinaction.science.uq.edu.au/edition1/?q=content/10-4-1-transformation-systems

Trigiano RN and Gray DJ, *Plant Tissue Concepts and Laboratory Exercises*, (Eds), CRC Press; available at http://pages.towson.edu/jsaunder/Saunders%20Publications/60.Use%20of%20protoplasts%20for%20plant%20improvement.pdf

Types of culture, Biotechnology 4U; available at http://www.biotechnology4u.com/plant_biotechnology_types_culture.html

Chapter 14 Enzyme Biotechnology

Enzyme Biotechnology, Molecular Plant Biotechnology.info; available at http://www.molecular-plant-biotechnology.info/enzyme-biotechnology/enzyme-biotechnology.htm

Enzyme-immobilization, Chemical Engineering Research Information Center; available at http://www.cheric.org/ippage/e/ipdata/2004/05/file/e200405-1101.pdf

Methods of Immobilization, Department of Chemistry and Chemical Biology at Renssalaer Polytechnic Institute; available at http://www.rpi.edu/dept/chem-eng/Biotech-Environ/IMMOB/methods.htm

Index